I0095833

When Pills Stop Working:

A Complete Guide To Advanced Solutions for Men

By Jay Richard

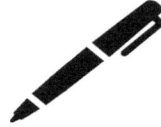

> "It is during our darkest moments
> that we must focus to see the light."

> **- Aristotle**

For information regarding bulk purchases, educational use, or special
editions, please contact the publisher at: info@seibroinc.com

This book is a work of original authorship.

Author: Jay Richard

Layout, design, and typography by Seibro Inc.

Published by Seibro Inc

Tampa, FL

Printed in the United States of America

First Edition, 2025

JayRichard.com

10 9 8 7 6 5 4 3 2 1

Copyright & Disclaimer

Content Warning: This book contains explicit discussions of sexual health, medical treatments, and clinical interventions related to erectile dysfunction. Content includes frank discussions of sexual function, intimate relationships, and medical procedures that some readers may find sensitive.

Medical Disclaimer: This book is intended solely for informational and educational purposes and should not be construed as medical advice or used as a substitute for professional medical consultation. The author is not a medical doctor and is not providing medical or therapeutic services through this publication. At times it may sound like the author is an expert or physician, but to be clear: he is not. The content represents personal opinions and information gathered from various sources, and all information should be independently verified.

Always consult with qualified healthcare providers, including urologists, primary care physicians, endocrinologists, or other specialists, before making any decisions regarding erectile dysfunction treatment, medication, or lifestyle changes. Individual circumstances vary significantly, and what may be appropriate for one person may not be suitable for another. Sexual health conditions can have complex underlying causes that require proper medical evaluation and diagnosis. If you are experiencing severe symptoms or have concerns about your sexual health, please consult with a healthcare professional promptly.

For additional resources and updates: www.jayrichard.com

Foreword

Erectile Dysfunction (ED) is a condition that affects millions of men worldwide, transcending cultural, geographic, and socioeconomic boundaries.

For many, it is more than just a physical ailment, it is a source of profound emotional and psychological distress, impacting self-esteem, relationships, and overall quality of life.
As a urologist, I have dedicated much of my career to helping men overcome this condition.

Over the years, I have witnessed significant advancements in medical science that have transformed the landscape of ED treatment. From oral medications to cutting-edge surgical procedures, the array of options available today allows for highly personalized care.

In this book, Jay explores the multifaceted nature of ED, delving into causes, treatments, and most importantly, one man's triumph over this condition. His courage to seek help and determination to regain control of his life were nothing short of inspiring.

This book serves as a resource for those struggling in silence, as well as for their loved ones and healthcare providers.
May it serve as a guide, a source of hope, and a reminder that no one must face this journey alone.

By William Figlesthaler, M.D., FACS

Table Of Contents

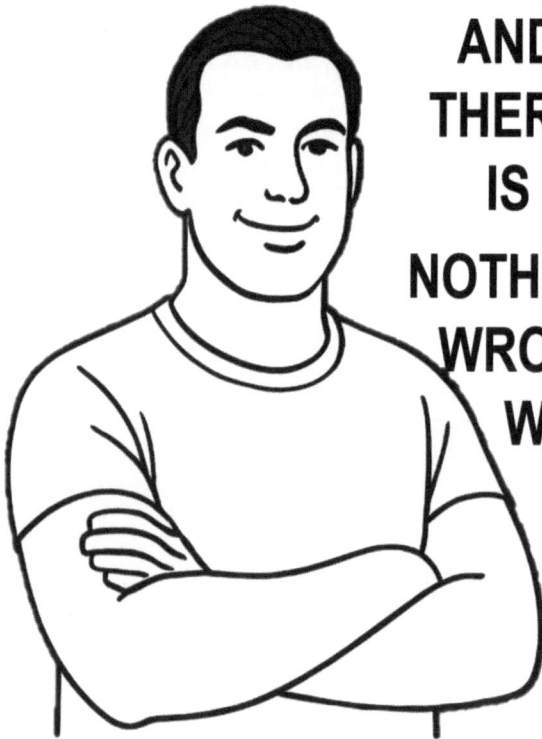

WE ARE SILENT SUFFERERS
BECAUSE WE ARE "*REAL MEN*"
AND THERE IS NOTHING WRONG WITH US

Introduction: The Journey Back To Confidence

At 3 am, the red digits on my bedside clock glowed mockingly in the darkness as I lay tangled in sweat-dampened sheets for the third night this week. The house creaked around me in the silence, punctuated only by my girlfriend's steady breathing beside me and the distant hum of the refrigerator downstairs. My fingers unconsciously traced the empty pill bottle on the nightstand, the plastic worn smooth from months of handling, the label's edges curled and faded.

The metallic taste of defeat coated my mouth as I finally admitted a truth I'd been avoiding for years: the pills had stopped working, and I was running out of options.

The weight of this realization settled in my chest like a stone, making each breath feel labored. Like millions of men worldwide, I was facing the reality that my sex life might be over, the thought hitting me with the same crushing finality as the sound of a door slamming shut.

I was wrong.

This book chronicles my journey from that dark moment to reclaiming not just my sexual function, but my confidence and joy in intimate relationships. If you're reading this, you're likely facing similar struggles—whether medications have lost their effectiveness, or you're wondering what comes next when traditional treatments fail.

You Are Not Alone

As you'll learn in the following chapters, erectile dysfunction affects an enormous number of men-far more than most people realize. These statistics don't even include the partners affected, essentially doubling the number of people dealing with ED's impact on their lives.

Yet, despite these overwhelming numbers, ED remains shrouded in silence. We are the "silent sufferers", men who feel isolated, embarrassed, and unsure where to turn when our most intimate function fails us.

Why This Book Exists

Most ED resources focus on pills and basic treatments. But what happens when those stop working? What do you do when you're facing the end of traditional options? This book fills that gap by providing a comprehensive guide to the next level of treatment: penile implant surgery.

Written by someone who lived through every aspect of this journey, this book offers:

- **Honest, personal experiences** from someone who's been where you are.
- **Practical medical information** about advanced treatment options.
- **Step-by-step guidance** through the decision-making process.
- **Real-world advice** about surgery, recovery, and life after treatment.
- **Financial guidance** for navigating costs and insurance.
- **Partner perspectives** often ignored in other resources.

What You'll Learn

This book will take you through the complete journey:

1. **Understanding ED**:

   What it really is and why it happens.

2. **When basic treatments fail**:

   Recognizing it's time for advanced options.

3. **Exploring penile implants**:

   Types, technology, and realistic expectations.

4. **Choosing the right surgeon**:

   Critical questions and evaluation criteria.

5. **Preparing for surgery**:

   What to expect before, during, and after.

6. **Financial planning**:

   Insurance, costs, and making it affordable.

7.Partner support

> How this affects relationships and how to navigate together.

8.Recovery and results:

> Real expectations and long-term outcomes.

A Message of Hope

Let me be clear from the start: there is hope for your currently, non-functioning penis.

The technology exists, the medical expertise is available, and thousands of men have successfully reclaimed their sexual lives through advanced treatments.

The journey may seem daunting, but you don't have to face it alone. This book will be your guide, providing the information, encouragement, and practical advice you need to make informed decisions about your sexual health.

Now Is The Time!

Why do we delay acting? Why don't we do everything we can to overcome ED now? Why don't we develop a plan to conquer this condition?

NOW IS THE TIME TO:

- Stop accepting a diminished quality of life!
- Explore all your options!
- Take control of your sexual health and confidence!

Let's make it your goal to become the lover you used to be, and perhaps even better than you were before.

Believe Me, You Can Be That Lover Again!

∞

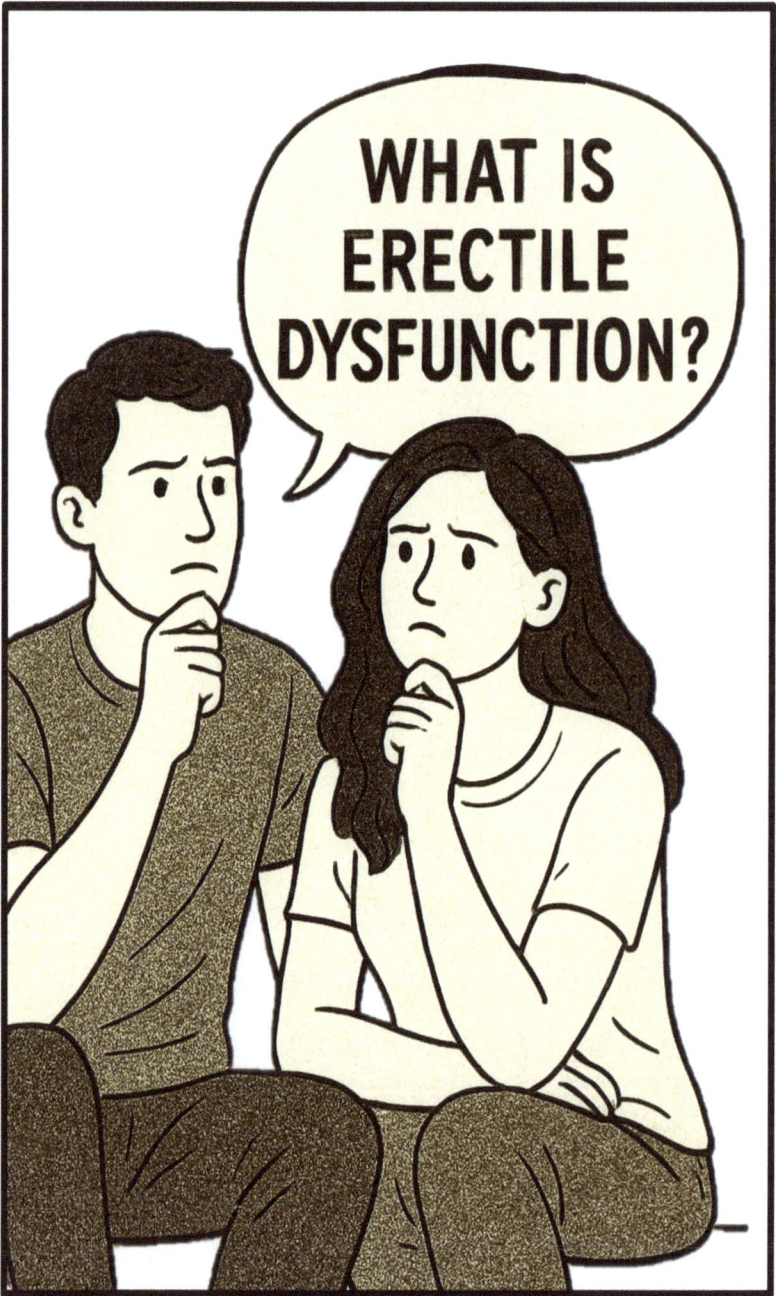

Chapter 1: Understanding Erectile Dysfunction

The Facts You Need to Know

L et me start with something that might surprise you: if you're reading this book: you're in remarkably good company.

I know that doesn't feel true when you're lying awake at 3 am wondering what's wrong with you, or when you're avoiding intimacy with your partner because you're terrified of another failure.

I've been exactly where you are now, and I want you to know that what you're experiencing has nothing to do with your worth as a man.

When my own struggle with erectile dysfunction began, I felt like I was the only guy in the world dealing with this nightmare. I was wrong-spectacularly wrong.

And once I learned the truth about how common this condition really is, everything changed. Not just my perspective, but my entire approach to getting my life back.

What Is Erectile Dysfunction?

Here's the medical definition: Erectile Dysfunction (ED) is the persistent inability to achieve or maintain an erection sufficient for satisfactory sexual intercourse.

But let me tell you what ED feels like from someone who lived with it for years.

ED isn't just about sex, though that's certainly part of it.

It's about lying next to your partner and feeling like a fraud.

It's about making excuses, avoiding situations, and slowly watching your confidence crumble.

It's about that sinking feeling when you realize that something as basic as your body's sexual response, something you never had to think about before, has suddenly become unreliable.

When I first started researching my condition, desperately Googling at 2 am, hoping to find some magic solution, I was overwhelmed by medical jargon and clinical descriptions that felt nothing like what I was experiencing.

Let me give you the real story in plain English.

First, and this took me way too long to accept: **ED is fundamentally a medical condition, not a mental weakness**. Yes, psychological factors can play a role, but for most of us, there are real, identifiable physical causes behind what's happening. You haven't lost your masculinity, and you haven't failed as a man. Your body is dealing with a medical issue that affects millions of guys.

Second, *ED* **tends to be progressive.** I wish someone had told me this upfront because I spent months hoping it would just go away on its own. Spoiler alert: it doesn't. In fact, it typically gets worse over time without proper medical intervention. The good news? That progression can be slowed or even reversed with the right treatment.

Third, and this is the most important thing I want you to understand, **ED is highly treatable.**
I mean *highly* treatable. We're not talking about some rare condition with limited options. There are multiple effective treatments available for nearly every case of ED. Yes, even yours.

The Numbers That Will Shock You (And Probably Comfort You Too)
Remember how I said you're in good company? Let me prove it with some statistics that genuinely floored me when I first learned them.
As you'll learn in the following chapters, more than half of all men between the ages of 40 and 70, specifically, 52 percent, experience some degree of ED during their lives. Read that again: **more than half**. But here's where it gets even more interesting. The prevalence follows what some doctors call the "rule of tens", roughly 10 percent of men per decade of life are affected. That means about 30 percent of men in their thirties experience some ED, 40 percent in their forties, 50 percent in their fifties, and so on. By the time men reach their sixties, approximately 60 percent are dealing with erectile difficulties.
This means that ED isn't just an *"older man's problem"* anymore. As I just mentioned, medical professionals are increasingly seeing this condition in men in their twenties and thirties,

largely due to lifestyle factors, stress, and health conditions that are becoming more common in younger generations.

In the United States alone, over 30 million men are currently affected by ED. Current projections show this number will grow to over 35 million by 2029. These aren't just numbers on a page, these represent millions of men who understand exactly what you're going through.

When we look globally, there are an estimated 300 million men worldwide currently experiencing ED which is projected to increase to 346 million by 2029.

Yet somehow, it remains the condition that nobody talks about.

Why? Because we've been conditioned to believe that real men don't have these problems, **which is complete nonsense**.

Understanding these numbers helped me realize that ED isn't some rare affliction, it's one of the most common health conditions affecting men. And that realization was the first step toward getting my life back.

Why This Happens to Us: The Real Culprits Behind ED

When I first developed ED, I went through what I now recognize as the classic stages of confusion and denial. First, I blamed stress. Then I blamed my age (even though I was in my early 60's). Then I blamed everything from my diet to my sleep schedule.

The truth is, erectile dysfunction rarely appears without a clear medical cause, and understanding these causes was crucial to finding the right treatment.

Cardiovascular Disease: The Silent Killer of Erections

Here's something your doctor might not have told you: your penis is basically a litmus test for your heart health. When blood vessels become damaged or narrowed due to conditions like high blood pressure, high cholesterol, or heart disease, the reduced blood flow affects your ability to get and maintain an erection.

Let me put this in perspective: getting an erection requires your body to rapidly pump about 7-8 times more blood to your penis than normal. If your cardiovascular system isn't firing on all cylinders, this whole process falls apart.

What really opened my eyes was learning that many heart doctors now consider ED an early warning sign of heart disease, sometimes showing up 3-5 years before you notice any heart problems. That hit home for me when I was diagnosed with atrial fibrillation during my own journey, which probably played a role in my condition.

Diabetes: The Double Whammy

Diabetes is particularly brutal when it comes to erectile function because it hits you from two directions, at least that's what some of my doctor friends explained to me.

First, it damages blood vessels throughout your body, including the ones essential for erections.

Second, it messes with your nerves, disrupting all those complex signals your body needs for normal sexual function.

Here's a statistic that absolutely floored me: anywhere from 60-75% of men with diabetes will experience some degree of ED, and erectile problems are often among the first signs that lead to a diabetes diagnosis.

If you're dealing with ED and haven't been tested for diabetes recently, I'd seriously consider making that a priority. Fortunately for me, diabetes wasn't the culprit, but it's definitely worth ruling out.

Other Potential Causes

Neurological Conditions: When the Wiring Gets Crossed

Your nervous system is like the electrical wiring for sexual function, it sends all the signals that start and maintain erections. Conditions like multiple sclerosis, Parkinson's disease, spinal cord injuries, and strokes can all throw a wrench into these processes. Even something as common as a herniated disc can sometimes mess with erectile function.

Hormonal Imbalances

Everyone talks about low testosterone (and yes, I discovered I had "Low T" too-more on that later), but hormonal causes of ED go way beyond that.

Through my research, I learned that thyroid problems, pituitary gland issues, and elevated prolactin levels can all impact sexual function.

Here's something interesting: being overweight can actually disrupt your hormone levels by converting testosterone into estrogen.

The Medication Trap

This one's particularly frustrating. Many common medications can interfere with erectile function as an unwanted side effect. My cardiologist warned me that certain blood pressure medications (especially diuretics and beta-blockers), some antidepressants (particularly SSRIs), antihistamines, and certain prostate medications can all contribute to ED.

The maddening part? Many of these medications are treating conditions that can cause ED in the first place. It's like a medical "catch 22": you need the medication for your health, but the medication creates the very problem you're trying to avoid.

Here's a perfect example from my own experience: when I first started exploring ED medications, my cardiologist told me they wouldn't work effectively if I took the blood thinner and beta-blocker he recommended for my atrial fibrillation. But I was so desperate to have a sex life that I made the incredibly stupid decision to keep taking my ED pills instead of the heart medications—literally risking a heart attack or stroke.

Somehow, I got through that period without a medical emergency, but looking back, it was one of the dumbest decisions I've ever made.

Lifestyle Factors: The Modern Epidemic

Lifestyle factors are becoming huge players in ED, especially for younger guys.

Smoking is a major villain because it damages blood vessels throughout your body—the chemicals in cigarettes literally poison the delicate blood vessels that serve your penis.

If you smoke and have ED, quitting is often the single most effective thing you can do to improve your situation.

Doctors have also told me that excessive drinking, not exercising regularly, poor sleep, chronic stress, and recreational drug use can all contribute to erectile problems.

The Psychological Component: It's Real, But Not What You Think

While physical causes account for most ED cases, psychological factors definitely play a role. Depression, anxiety, chronic stress, relationship problems, and performance anxiety can all interfere with sexual function.

But here's the cruel irony: ED itself often causes these psychological issues, creating a vicious cycle that's incredibly hard to break without professional help.

When to Stop Hoping It Will Go Away and Get Help

I waited way too long to seek help.

Way too Long!

I kept thinking that if I just reduced stress, exercised more, ate better, or tried some supplement I found online, things would magically return to normal.

I was wrong, and that delay cost me months of frustration and damaged relationships.

You should talk to a healthcare provider if you've been experiencing ED symptoms for more than two to three months. While occasional erectile difficulties are totally normal, persistent issues lasting several months suggest something underlying that needs attention.

I've been told you should seek immediate medical attention if:

- You experience sudden onset of ED, especially if you're younger or have no obvious risk factors.
- ED occurs alongside chest pain, dizziness, shortness of breath, or unusual fatigue.
- ED begins to significantly affect your quality of life, relationships, or emotional well-being.

If you suspect medications you're taking might be contributing to erectile problems, discuss this with your healthcare provider immediately.

Don't stop taking prescribed medications without medical supervision, but don't suffer in silence either.

Understanding Your Treatment Options: From Pills to Possibilities

Later in the book, I'll walk you through the multiple treatment options that exist, ranging from simple lifestyle changes to advanced surgical interventions. When I first learned about this spectrum of treatments, it gave me hope for the first time in months.

First-Line Treatments: Most guys start with oral medications like Viagra, Cialis, and Levitra. These work by enhancing blood flow to the penis during sexual arousal. But here's what those commercials don't tell you: these pills only work for about 60-70% of men who try them. They also have limitations including potential side effects, drug interactions, and the need for advance planning.

Second-Line Treatments: When oral medications aren't cutting it, options include penile injection therapy (with success rates of 60-80%), vacuum erection devices, herbs, urethral suppositories, and newer experimental treatments.

Third-Line Treatments: When conservative treatments fail, penile implants represent the most effective and reliable treatment for ED, which is why they're the focus of this book. These surgically implanted devices provide the highest patient satisfaction rates, with over 90% of men reporting satisfaction with their results.

Why Pills Stop Working: The Frustrating Reality

If you're reading this book, you've likely experienced the frustration of ED medications that once worked but have become less effective or stopped working entirely. This happened to me, and understanding why helped me move forward with confidence.

Some men develop tolerance to ED medications, and drug interactions can interfere with effectiveness as we age and require additional medications for other health conditions.

The Path Forward: Your Journey Starts Here

While dealing with ED can be frustrating and emotionally challenging, it doesn't reflect your worth as a man or as a partner. If oral medications and other basic treatments have failed, don't lose hope.

Advanced options like penile implants offer the possibility of restored sexual function and renewed confidence.

The following chapters will guide you through these options and help you make the best decisions for your situation.

Most importantly, don't let embarrassment or shame prevent you from seeking the help you need and deserve.
You've already taken the first step by picking up this book.
Now let's figure out how to get your life back.

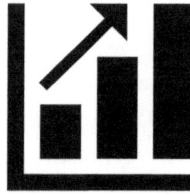

DID YOU KNOW?

Over 30 million American men experience erectile dysfunction

You are not alone in this journey!

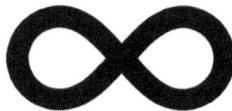

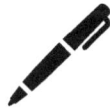

"The greatest revolution of our generation
is the discovery that human beings,
by changing the inner attitudes of their minds,
can change the outer aspects of their lives."

- William James

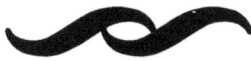

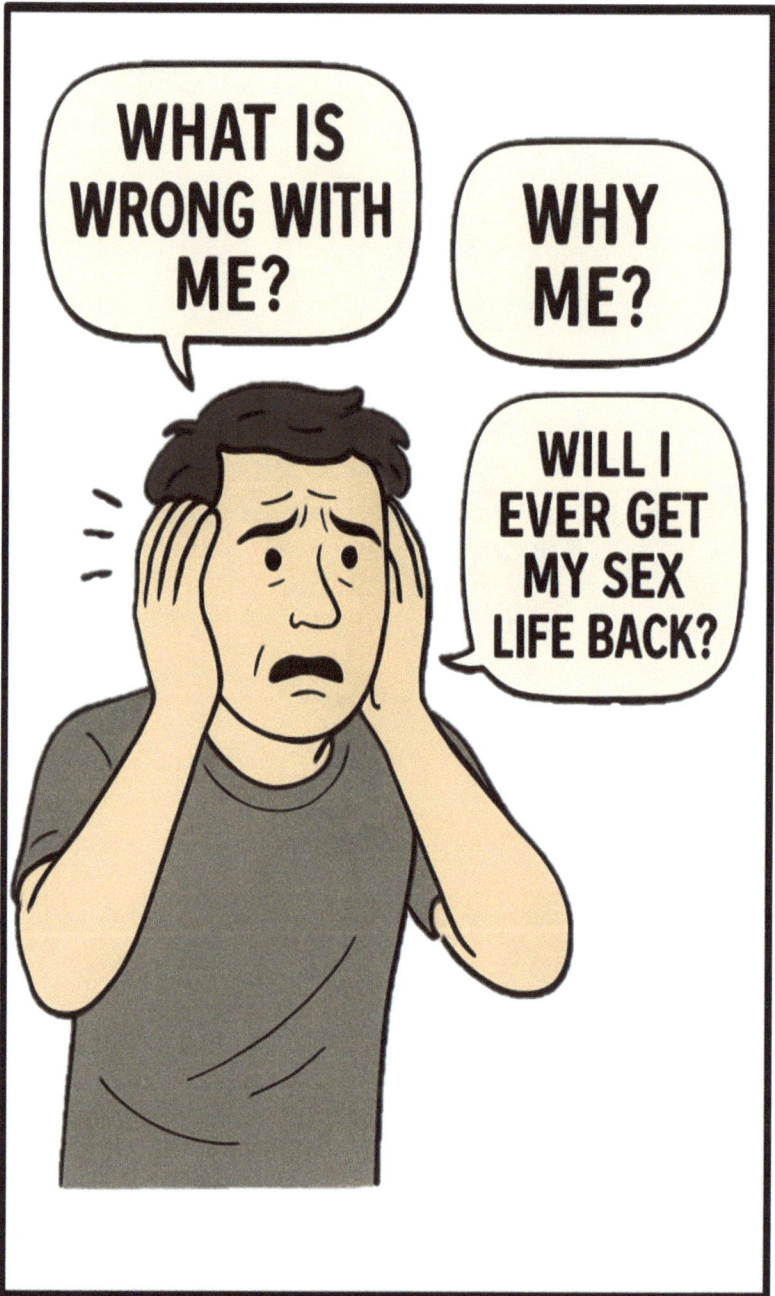

Chapter 2: My Personal Journey
From Denial to Decision

The first time it happened; I dismissed it as a fluke. Maybe I was tired, maybe I'd had too much to drink, maybe it was just one of those things that occasionally happens to every man. The second time, I made excuses. The third time, I began to worry. By the time it became a pattern, denial was no longer possible, but I clung to hope anyway, convincing myself that if I just waited long enough, things would return to normal.

It never did.

What followed was a journey that took me from stubborn denial through desperate attempts at quick fixes, from humiliating failures to crushing loneliness, and finally to a decision that would transform my life.

If you're reading this chapter, you're likely somewhere on a similar path. My hope is that sharing my story will help you feel less alone and perhaps find the courage to act sooner than I did.

When My Body Betrayed Me

Looking back, I realize I was fortunate that my introduction to erectile dysfunction happened gradually rather than suddenly. At first, the problems were intermittent enough that I could rationalize them away. I was in my sixties, in excellent physical health, and had always considered myself sexually confident. The idea that my body might be failing me in such a fundamental way seemed impossible.

The progression was insidious.

What began as occasional difficulties became more frequent problems, and eventually, reliable function became the exception rather than the rule.

Each incident chipped away at my confidence, creating a growing sense of dread around intimate situations. I found myself hoping that romantic evenings wouldn't lead to sexual expectations, and when they did, I approached them with anxiety rather than anticipation.

The psychological impact proved as devastating as the physical problem. Sex had always been a source of pleasure and connection, but it gradually became a minefield of potential embarrassment and failure.

I began avoiding situations that, even though I was married at that time, might lead to intimacy, preferring the safety of loneliness to the risk of sexual humiliation.

I need to be honest about something that's painful to share but important for you to understand: my marriage didn't survive my struggle with ED, and I'm not entirely sure it would have even with successful treatment.

I'll never forget the evening that crystallized my isolation.

It was a Tuesday night in March, and I finally worked up the courage to discuss our sexual problems with my then wife.

"We have a problem," I told her, hoping for understanding and partnership in facing this challenge together.

Her response was swift and unambiguous: "No, *WE* don't have a problem. *YOU* have a problem."

Her words revealed something that went deeper than just her reaction to my erectile dysfunction. It showed me that she didn't see us as a team facing life's challenges together.

Those words stung more than any physical pain could have.

In that instant, I realized I would be facing this challenge alone, without the support of the person closest to me. What should have been a team effort became a solitary struggle, made infinitely more difficult by the lack of understanding from the one person whose support I needed most.

Looking back, I realize that our marriage had been struggling in other ways, and ED became the catalyst that exposed existing cracks rather than creating new ones. The lack of emotional support when I was most vulnerable, the complete unwillingness to discuss the issue as partners, and her attitude that this was entirely my burden to bear alone made me realize we had fundamental differences in how we approached the marriage itself.

Later, the divorce process was complicated by the timing, right in the middle of my ED struggles. I found myself dealing with both the loss of sexual function and the loss of my marriage simultaneously. Some nights, I couldn't tell which was causing more pain.

But here's what I learned: if your partner isn't willing to support you through health challenges, that tells you something crucial about your relationship's foundation. My current girlfriend's completely different response---curiosity, support, and treating this as something we'd figure out together---showed me what a true partnership looks like.

I share this not to discourage you, but to help you understand that while ED can stress relationships, it often reveals the true nature of your partnership rather than destroying an otherwise strong bond.

The Desperate Search for Solutions

Like most men facing erectile dysfunction, I began with the most obvious solution: pills.

Viagra had been a revolutionary development, and surely it would solve my problem quickly and easily. (Later, Cialis became my pill of choice).

I approached my family doctor, who happened to be a friend, though even this familiar relationship, I couldn't entirely overcome the embarrassment of discussing such an intimate issue.

In the beginning, the pills worked most of the time, which kept alive the hope that they might work consistently.

But their unpredictability created its own torture.

I never knew whether any given encounter would be successful or disappointing, which meant that every intimate moment carried the weight of uncertainty. Sometimes the medication worked reasonably well, giving me false hope that my problems were resolving. Other times, despite identical circumstances and timing, nothing would happen.

I experimented with different medications, dosages, and timing. I tried herbal supplements, combinations of treatments, and various lifestyle modifications.

Each approach offered the promise of success but delivered only inconsistent results. The pattern of hope followed by disappointment became more psychologically damaging than complete failure might have been.

As my marriage deteriorated under the strain of sexual dysfunction and lack of emotional support, I found myself facing the prospect of divorce.

The combination of my withdrawal from intimacy, my wife's unwillingness to treat this as a shared challenge, and the growing tension around our sexual relationship created a destructive cycle that we never managed to break.

Navigating My New Single Life with a Secret

Re-entering the dating world as a single man with unreliable sexual function presented challenges I had never anticipated.

Every new relationship carried the potential for romantic progression, which meant eventual sexual expectations. The anxiety this created was almost overwhelming.

I found myself developing elaborate strategies to avoid sexual situations while still maintaining the appearance of normal social and romantic behavior.

One approach involved deliberately pursuing women I wasn't strongly attracted to.

If I didn't feel genuine desire, I reasoned, we wouldn't progress to sexual situations where my dysfunction would be exposed.

How dumb was this thinking?

This strategy allowed me to maintain social connections and the appearance of an active dating life while avoiding the risk of sexual failure. However, it also meant accepting relationships that lacked passion or genuine connection.

Another tactic involved ending potentially promising relationships before they could progress to physical intimacy. I became skilled at identifying when a relationship might be heading toward sexual expectations and would find reasons to withdraw before that point.

I convinced myself that this preserved both my dignity and theirs, since they would never discover my secret shame.

These avoidance behaviors might have protected my immediate ego, but they came at an enormous cost.

I was essentially removing myself from the possibility of genuine intimate connection, choosing loneliness over the risk of embarrassment. I was missing opportunities for love, partnership, and happiness because I was too afraid to be vulnerable about my medical condition.

The Fantasy That Became a Nightmare

One evening stands out as a perfect example of how erectile dysfunction could transform even the most promising situation into crushing disappointment.

I had been flirting with an attractive woman at a cocktail party, and the chemistry between us was obvious to everyone present. When she needed a ride home, I offered eagerly, sensing that the evening might lead somewhere special.

On the way, we needed to stop at my house to let my dog out. She noticed my pool and spa and asked if she could go swimming. What happened next seemed like the fulfillment of every man's fantasy.

She undressed unselfconsciously in my kitchen and slipped into the pool, beckoning for me to join her. The foreplay in the pool and spa was incredible, and I felt more optimistic about my prospects than I had in months. (In anticipation, I had taken medication earlier in the evening, hoping for a possibility of romance and was getting prepared if it happened).

But when the moment came to move beyond foreplay, my body refused to cooperate.

Despite the perfect setup, the medication, and my genuine attraction to this woman, I couldn't achieve an erection.

The harder I tried to will my body to respond, the more obvious my failure became.

What should have been a night of passion became an exercise in damage control.

Fortunately, I had learned alternative ways to provide satisfaction, and I was able to bring her to multiple orgasms using manual techniques. She seemed genuinely pleased and fell asleep contentedly beside me.

From her perspective, the evening had been successful, but for me, it highlighted everything I was missing.

While I could provide pleasure to my partner, I was denied the intimacy and connection of actual intercourse.

She left early the next morning, clearly embarrassed by the previous night's spontaneity (she had too much to drink), and I never heard from her again.

Even though the encounter hadn't been a complete disaster, it reinforced my growing conviction that my sexual dysfunction was stealing away opportunities for genuine connection and meaningful relationships.

The Psychological Prison

Living with unpredictable erectile dysfunction created a psychological prison that extended far beyond the bedroom. The fear of sexual failure continued to color every aspect of my thinking about relationships and self-worth.

I found myself constantly analyzing my body's responses, looking for signs that function might be returning or confirmation that it was getting worse.

The unpredictability was perhaps the cruelest aspect of the condition.

If I had been completely unable to achieve erections, I could have adapted to that reality and focused entirely on alternative forms of intimacy.

Instead, the occasional success kept alive the hope that normal function might return, making each failure feel like a fresh disappointment rather than an expected outcome.

My sexual repertoire became severely limited.

I could achieve penetration only in the missionary position, and even then, I had perhaps sixty to ninety seconds before losing the erection.

This meant I had to climax quickly, which felt selfish but was necessary to achieve any satisfaction at all for me. The pressure to perform rapidly made sex feel rushed and mechanical rather than intimate and connected.

I dated one woman at this time that called me "The 30 Second Man".

Why? Only because of my quick 30 second orgasm that came out of fear that I could not hold my erection any longer.

I began to question my worth as a partner and wonder who would want to be in a relationship with someone who couldn't perform sexually.

The constant worry about performance invaded my thoughts even in non-sexual situations. Dating continued to be fraught with anxiety because every encounter carried the potential for sexual expectations and subsequent failure.

A Brutal Truth

One relationship provided particularly stark insight into how my erectile dysfunction was affecting my partners, even when I thought I was managing the situation reasonably well.

I had been seeing a woman long-distance for nearly a year, spending every other weekend together. Our relationship seemed solid, and I believed our sexual connection was adequate given my limitations.

I was completely unprepared to discover that she was maintaining a purely sexual relationship with another man in her hometown on the weekends she was home "alone."

As a mutual friend told me later (my girlfriend had shared her reasoning with her) it was very simple: "Sex with him (me) just isn't that good. He needs a complete overhaul in that department."

This explanation was devastating in its honesty, but very true.

While her infidelity was unacceptable and ended our relationship, I had to acknowledge that her assessment of my sexual performance was painfully accurate.

I was indeed a limited lover, capable of providing some satisfaction through manual techniques but unable to offer the full intimate experience that most women desired and deserved.

This revelation forced me to confront the reality that my erectile dysfunction wasn't just my private struggle. It was significantly impacting my partners in ways I hadn't fully understood or acknowledged.

Women were either accepting unsatisfying sexual relationships with me or, as in this case, seeking satisfaction elsewhere while maintaining the relationship for its other benefits.

The Moment of Truth

The turning point in my journey came during a quiet Sunday morning when I was reflecting on the direction of my life, and not happy with it..

As I noted earlier, I was actively avoiding dating and intimate situations, essentially removing myself from one of life's greatest sources of joy and connection.

I had accepted isolation as preferable to the risk of sexual failure, but in doing so, I was missing opportunities for love, partnership, and happiness.

My choice seemed obvious: between taking action to reclaim my life or accepting a future characterized by loneliness, missed opportunities, and gradually diminishing hope.

When I framed the decision in those terms, the path forward became much clearer.

Several realizations converged to create this moment of clarity. I acknowledged that erectile dysfunction doesn't improve on its own and that the years I had spent hoping for spontaneous recovery had only resulted in worsening symptoms and increasing psychological damage.

I recognized that I was too young to surrender this aspect of my life, with potentially decades ahead of me. I finally understood that this was fundamentally a medical problem rather than a character flaw or failure of willpower.

Most importantly, I realized that effective solutions had to exist if I had the courage to pursue them.

My happiness and fulfillment mattered enough to justify taking some risks to improve my situation. I deserved to have a fulfilling intimate life, and I had the power to make that happen.

Discovering Hope Through Research

Once I committed to finding a real solution, I began extensive research into treatment options beyond the basic medications that had failed me.

This educational process proved transformative because it revealed that my pill failures didn't mean I was out of options. Instead, I was simply ready to move to the next level of treatment.

I began exploring in more detail injection therapy, vacuum devices, speculative tools, and ultimately surgical options.

Each level of treatment seemed to offer better and more consistent results than the previous one.

Most importantly, I began educating myself about urologists who specialize specifically in sexual medicine.

These physicians possess knowledge and treatment options that go far beyond what most general practitioners can offer.

The existence of specialists dedicated to treating conditions like mine made me realize that I wasn't facing an insurmountable problem but rather a medical condition with established treatment protocols.

This research phase was crucial because it transformed my sense of hopelessness into cautious optimism.

I began to understand that modern medicine offered sophisticated solutions for men in my situation, and that thousands of men had successfully overcome similar challenges.

Finding Unexpected Support

One of the most encouraging aspects of moving forward was discovering that I wasn't as alone as I had felt. Support came from several unexpected sources, each contributing to my growing confidence about pursuing advanced treatment.

For example, during a routine visit with my urologist, Dr. Figlesthaler, known affectionately as "Dr. Fig", I asked the question that had been weighing on my mind: "Is there anything new in the "pills arena", or something that will help my ED go away?"

It was here that Dr. Fig stated that since I had tried most everything, there was one option left that could work for me: penile implant surgery.

I had heard about it and had not pursued it as I'm a "chicken" and did want to do anything that might "hurt."

Wow, was I naïve!

He introduced me to his staff, and I was totally blown away when they treated me and my condition as a routine medical issue rather than something unusual.

This normalization of what felt like an overwhelming decision helped reduce my anxiety and build confidence in the treatment process.

Next, after church one day during a casual conversation with a guy I had sat next to for years, I mentioned that I was considering "man surgery" and would not be at church next week. He asked what the heck is "man surgery" several times, and to get him off my back, I finally told him it was known as penile implant surgery, which I was sure he had never heard of. To my surprise, he quickly shared that he had undergone the same procedure three years earlier.

"Best decision I ever made," he said with a knowing smile. And he was 88 years old and still going strong sexually with his wife. That conversation helped transform my anxiety into anticipation and showed me that successful men around me had quietly solved this problem.

Then I found several online communities of men facing similar challenges provided additional perspective and practical advice.

Reading about other men's experiences, both their struggles and their successes, helped me understand that my journey was part of a larger pattern of men reclaiming their sexual health through modern medical interventions.

The Decision That Changed Everything

After months of research, soul-searching, and careful consideration, I made the decision to proceed with penile implant surgery.

This wasn't a choice I made lightly or quickly, but once I committed to this path, I felt a sense of relief and anticipation that had been absent from my life for years.

The decision required me to overcome several psychological barriers.

I had to accept that my natural erectile function would be permanently compromised and that mechanical assistance would be necessary for the rest of my life.

I had to acknowledge that surgery, even minor surgery, carried some risks.

I had to commit to a recovery period and the learning curve associated with using an implanted device.

However, these concerns paled in comparison to the potential benefits. The prospect of reliable erectile function, freedom from performance anxiety, and the ability to engage in intimate relationships without fear of failure outweighed any concerns about the surgical process or recovery period.

Looking back, I wish I had made this decision years earlier. The time I spent hoping for spontaneous improvement, trying ineffective treatments, and avoiding intimate situations represented years of unnecessarily diminished quality of life.

Once I committed to surgical treatment, I began to feel hopeful about my future in ways that had been impossible during the long struggle with unreliable erectile function.

Lessons for Others

My journey from denial through desperation to decision taught me several important lessons that might help other men facing similar challenges.

The most crucial insight is that delaying treatment typically makes the problem worse, both physically and psychologically. Erectile dysfunction doesn't improve with time, and the psychological damage from repeated failures becomes increasingly difficult to overcome.

The importance of education cannot be overstated. Understanding my condition and learning about available treatments reduced my fear and built confidence in my eventual decision.

Knowledge helped me realize that I wasn't facing an unusual or insurmountable problem but rather a common medical condition with established solutions.

Support from others who had faced similar challenges proved invaluable. Whether from medical professionals, friends who had undergone similar procedures, or online communities of men dealing with erectile dysfunction, connecting with others reduced my sense of isolation and provided practical guidance for moving forward.

Perhaps most importantly, I learned that acting requires courage, but the courage to seek help is far easier to summon than the courage required to continue living with the problem. The anticipation of treatment is typically worse than the reality, and the benefits of successful treatment extend far beyond the restoration of sexual function.

Moving Forward with Hope

If you see yourself in my story, take heart.

The feelings of frustration, embarrassment, and isolation you're experiencing are temporary. The sense of hopelessness that may seem overwhelming right now can be replaced with optimism and anticipation. With proper medical treatment, you can reclaim not just your sexual function but your confidence and joy in intimate relationships.

The decision to pursue advanced treatment like penile implants represents a choice to stop accepting diminished quality of life and start taking control of your health and happiness. It's a decision to invest in your future rather than simply hoping that your past problems will somehow resolve themselves.

The journey from denial to decision was the most difficult part of my entire experience.

Once I committed to getting help, everything else fell into place.

The path forward became clear, hope replaced despair, and I began to envision a future that included the intimate relationships I had been missing.

That transformation is available to you as well, but it begins with the decision to stop accepting your current situation and start pursuing the life you deserve.

The following chapters will guide you through the practical aspects of exploring your options, making informed decisions, and navigating the treatment process successfully.

The most important step, however, is the one you take right now: the decision to believe that your situation can improve and that you deserve to be happy. ∞

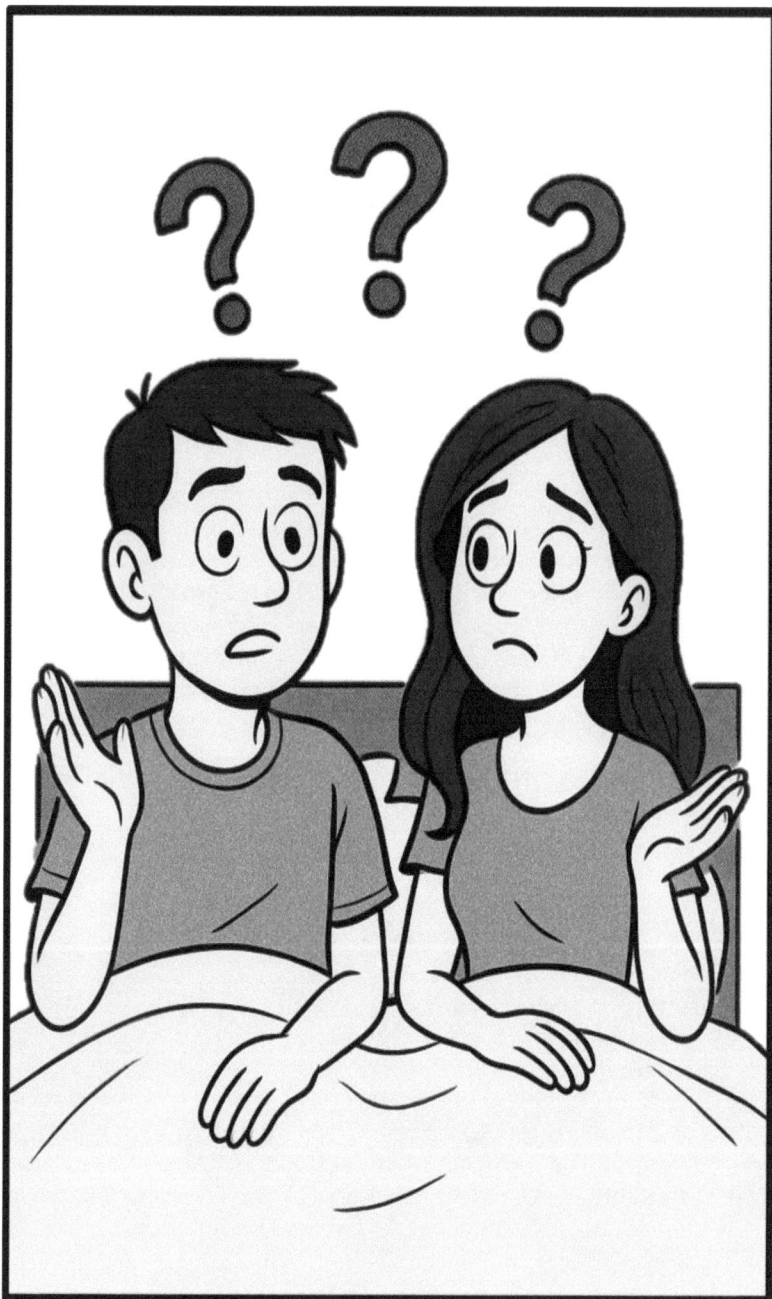

Chapter 3: When Pills Stop Working
Exploring Your Options

The morning after another failed attempt with a 100mg Viagra—the highest dose available—I sat at my kitchen table with my laptop, desperately searching for answers. My girlfriend had gone to work early, sparing us both the awkwardness of discussing another disappointment. Three years of relying on the little blue pill, and now even that lifeline seemed gone. If you're reading this book, you've likely discovered what I was forced to confront that devastating morning: pills aren't magic bullets, and even when they work initially, their effectiveness can fade over time.

This reality felt crushing, like watching my last hope disappear. But here's what became clear during those dark hours of internet searching: this wasn't the end of my options, it was the beginning of exploring treatments that could work better and more reliably than pills ever had.

My journey from pill failure to renewed sexual function required understanding why my medications had betrayed me, recognizing what alternatives existed, and finding the courage to pursue more advanced treatments.

If only someone had explained why my medications stopped working instead of leaving me to figure it out through trial and error. This chapter will guide you through that process as I experienced it, helping you see that what feels like a dead end is a doorway to better solutions.

Understanding Why My Pills Betrayed Me

The first time a Viagra failed after working for several years, I assumed I'd done something wrong.

Maybe the timing was off, maybe I'd eaten too much beforehand, maybe stress from work had interfered with the medication's effectiveness. When failures became more frequent over the following months, the excuses became harder to maintain, and a terrible realization set in as the treatment that once offered hope was no longer reliable.

Through my desperate research, I learned that my progression followed predictable patterns that had nothing to do with willpower or technique.

My research confirmed what I'd learned about ED being a progressive condition---the underlying causes typically worsen over time, as we discussed earlier.

In my case, the cardiovascular issues that may have caused my initial ED continued to accumulate. The arteries serving my penis were becoming increasingly narrowed, eventually reaching a point where oral medications could no longer overcome the circulation problems.

My research helped me understand that my body had probably developed tolerance to ED medications, like how people become accustomed to caffeine. The same 50mg or 100mg dose that once produced reliable erections had gradually become less effective. When I'd increased to 100mg, it worked for a while, but eventually even that maximum dose became insufficient.

Perhaps most insidiously, my repeated pill failures had also created a psychological cycle that made the medications even less effective. Each disappointment increased my anxiety about the next encounter, and this performance anxiety directly interfered with erectile function. I found myself approaching intimate situations with dread rather than anticipation, which virtually guaranteed poor results regardless of medication timing or dosage.

The cruel irony was that the more desperately I needed the pills to work, the less likely they became to provide reliable results. This cycle had transformed me from someone who once felt sexually confident into a man who avoided intimate situations entirely, preferring the safety of isolation to the risk of another humiliating failure.

Discovering the Treatment Ladder

One of the most important concepts I learned during my research was that erectile dysfunction treatment exists on a spectrum, with each level offering progressively better results for men who don't respond to simpler approaches.

Pills represented just the first rung on this ladder, and their failure simply meant I was ready to climb higher.

I learned that second-line treatments offered significantly better success rates for many rather than oral medications, often providing reliable results for men who found pills completely ineffective.

These approaches bypassed some of the limitations that made pills unreliable, working through different mechanisms to achieve the same goal of increasing blood flow to the penis.

My Experience with Injection Therapy

I tried penile injection therapy as it seemed to be a popular common and effective second-line treatment.

The idea of injecting medication directly into my penis sounded terrifying initially, but I was desperate enough to try anything. The medication was designed to bypass my digestive system and act directly on the blood vessels within the penis, creating erections that were often firmer and more reliable than what pills ever provided.

I tried this at a clinic that was advertised on our local cable channel. The injection process itself was simpler than I'd imagined. Using a very fine needle like those used by diabetics, the nurse injected a small amount of Trimix into the side of my penis. The injection took just a few seconds, and the discomfort was minimal and brief.

The medication worked.

Within ten minutes, I had an erection that was hard as a rock, firmer than anything I'd achieved lately with pills.

But several problems quickly became apparent. The timing felt too delayed and clinical for me. By the time the erection arrived, the spontaneous moment would have passed. Worse, my penis ended up bruised from the injection, and the whole experience felt too uncomfortable and unnatural for me to want to try again.

Many men find injections provide the reliability and confidence that pills never delivered.

But for me, the trade-offs weren't acceptable.

My Disappointing Experience with Vacuum Devices

I also tried a vacuum erection device, which works through purely mechanical means.

Essentially this device uses suction to draw blood into the penis, creating an erection that's maintained using a constriction ring placed at the base of the penis.

I had a friend that swore by this option, so I figured what the heck, I'll give it a try.

Medicare provided a medical-grade vacuum, and I hoped it might offer a solution without the discomfort of injections.

While the device was effective at achieving erections suitable for intercourse, I found it cumbersome and unnatural feeling. The erections produced felt less firm than natural erections, and the process interrupted spontaneity in ways that I found unacceptable.

But the vacuum approach offered certain advantages, particularly since I could use it safely with my blood thinner medications without worrying about drug interactions.

And, another benefit, there were no ongoing medication costs.

However, the mechanical nature of the process made intimate encounters feel clinical rather than romantic, which defeated the purpose for me.

Herbs

Before accepting that prescription medication might be failing me, I dove deep into the world of herbal supplements. I tried everything from horny goat weed and ginseng to L-arginine and yohimbe bark extract. The appeal was obvious: natural solutions without the side effects and prescription requirements of pharmaceutical drugs.

Initially, many of these herbs seemed promising and even worked for me to a certain degree.

Combinations of ginseng and L-arginine would work remarkably well for the first few days or weeks, giving me hope that I'd found my natural solution. The effects felt more gradual and organic than pills—less like flipping a switch and more like rekindling something that had been dormant.

But without fail, every herbal remedy for me followed the same disappointing pattern: what worked brilliantly at first would gradually lose effectiveness, leaving me constantly searching for the next combination or higher dosage.

In one particularly frustrating episode, I doubled up on a potent yohimbe-based formula, convinced that more would restore the initial effectiveness.

Instead, I ended up with a painful urinary tract infection (UTI) that required an urgent doctor visit and a course of antibiotics to clear up.

That UTI was a wake-up call about the risks of self-medicating with "natural" substances that can have very real physiological effects.

Each of these second-line treatments had taught me something important: they might work mechanically, but they all felt artificial and interrupted the natural flow of intimacy that my girlfriend and I were trying to restore.

The Testosterone Wild Goose Chase

Before I fully accepted that my ED was primarily vascular, I spent several months convinced that low testosterone was my real problem. The appeal was obvious---if I could just get my T levels up, maybe everything would return to normal naturally.

My primary care doctor ordered the blood work, and sure enough, my testosterone was a little below the normal range.

"Here's my answer." I thought. "Fix the testosterone, fix the problem."

I tried testosterone gel first. Every morning, I'd apply this clear gel to my shoulders, then spend the day wondering if I felt more energetic, more sexual, more like my younger self. The placebo effect was strong initially, I convinced myself I felt better for the first six weeks.

But my ED didn't improve. My energy did increase somewhat, and my mood was better, but when it came to sexual function, nothing changed. My doctor increased the dose. We tried injections. We added other medications to boost my body's natural production.

After many months of optimizing my testosterone to levels higher than I'd had in my twenties, I had to face the truth: this was not my solution. My ED had other causes that testosterone could not fix.

The most frustrating part was how much hope I'd invested in this approach. I'd read countless forum posts from men claiming testosterone therapy had "cured" their ED. I'd convinced myself that I just needed to find the right dose, the right delivery method, the right combination.

What I learned is that while low testosterone can contribute to ED, especially reduced libido, it's rarely the primary cause in men with vascular or nerve-related problems. For me, testosterone therapy became a several months detour that delayed pursuing treatments that could help.

If you're considering testosterone therapy, by all means try it---but don't let it become an excuse to avoid addressing the real causes of your ED.

The Search for the Next "Magic Bullet"

The failure of testosterone therapy hit me harder than I expected. I'd invested so much hope in that approach, convinced that optimizing my hormone levels would unlock the solution I'd been seeking. When it didn't work, I found myself back at square one, but now with even less confidence in conventional treatments.

This is when I entered what I now recognize as the "desperation phase" of my ED journey. Having exhausted first-line oral medications, second line treatments, and experienced the disappointment of testosterone therapy, I became increasingly drawn to newer, more experimental treatments. The internet was full of promising-sounding approaches that claimed to "regenerate" or "restore" natural function, and part of me wanted to believe these cutting-edge treatments might be the answer that traditional medicine couldn't provide.

I researched all the options below but didn't try any of them. They didn't seem right for my situation for one reason or another. If you're interested in exploring these options, I suggest you verify this information and discuss it with your medical advisor to see if they might make sense for you.

Platelet-Rich Plasma (PRP) -The "P-Shot"

This treatment involves drawing your blood, concentrating the platelets, then injecting them into penile tissue with the goal of promoting regeneration and improving blood flow. The appeal was obvious using my own blood meant minimal risk, and "natural regeneration" sounded better than mechanical devices.

However, when I researched the evidence, most studies were small, and results were inconsistent. With no guarantee of success and potentially requiring multiple sessions, it felt like it could be an expensive gamble.

Low-Intensity Shock Wave Therapy (LIESWT)

This uses acoustic waves to supposedly stimulate blood vessel growth in penile tissue. The safety profile seemed excellent, and the treatment was non-invasive-6-12 sessions over several months, 20 minutes each.

But the results remained unpredictable. While some men benefited, there was no way to know who would respond, and even advocates admitted benefits might be temporary. It looked to me that the cost of multiple sessions could add up quickly did not appeal to me.

Stem Cell Therapy

The theory was compelling, harvest stem cells from my fat tissue and inject them into penile tissue to regenerate blood vessels and nerves. Some marketing materials promised to "reverse" ED by "harnessing your body's natural healing power."

The clinical evidence, however, seemed years away from proving efficacy. Most studies were preliminary. With a substantial financial investment required for the full protocol, it seemed like an expensive experiment.

Gene Therapy

Academic centers were researching gene therapy approaches, though still in early phases. While fascinating from a scientific perspective, the timeline for clinical availability again seemed years away. This might help future generations, but I needed a solution now.

The Bottom Line on "Magic Bullets"

What struck me about all these alternatives was how speculative they remained. The clinics offering them were honest about being "cutting-edge" and "innovative," but what I needed was reliability. I'd already spent years hoping treatments would work and dealing with disappointment. These newer treatments offered more uncertainty, not less.

Recognizing When It Was Time for Advanced Treatment

After failing with pills, injections, vacuum devices, and ruling out the speculative treatments, I had to face reality. Several patterns indicated that more advanced intervention was necessary for me.

My fear of needles had prevented consistent use of injection therapy, even when it worked mechanically. The dosages required were at the higher end of the recommended range, and I worried about developing scar tissue from repeated injections. The physical discomfort and psychological barriers made injection therapy impractical for long-term use.

The vacuum device, while effective at producing erections, created relationship stress that undermined its benefits. My girlfriend had tried to be supportive, but the mechanical nature of the process made our intimate encounters feel clinical rather than romantic. The interruption of spontaneity that characterized most second-line treatments was creating new problems to replace the ones I was trying to solve.

Quality of life considerations became paramount in my evaluation. Second-line treatments felt burdensome, unreliable, and incompatible with my lifestyle and relationship goals. I was reaching a point where I desired a permanent solution that didn't require ongoing medication, planning, or mechanical devices.

The emotional toll was also becoming unsustainable. Each failed treatment attempt increased my anxiety about sexual performance and created additional relationship strain.

My girlfriend and I were both walking on eggshells around intimacy, which was exactly the opposite of what we were trying to achieve.

The Promise of Third-Line Treatment

When conservative treatments proved inadequate for me, penile implants represented the most effective and reliable solution for erectile dysfunction.

My research showed that this surgical option provided the highest patient satisfaction rates of any ED treatment, with over ninety percent of men reporting satisfaction with their results.

More importantly, implants offered the reliability and spontaneity that pills, and other treatments could not provide for me.

Understanding penile implants required recognizing that these devices completely replace your natural erectile mechanism with a mechanical system that you control.

Once the implant is in place, natural erections become impossible, but the device provides reliable erections whenever desired. I was becoming increasingly comfortable with this trade-off between natural function and mechanical reliability.

Modern implants were sophisticated medical devices that had been refined over decades of development.

They were designed to be durable, reliable, and as natural, feeling as possible. The surgery required for implantation had become a routine procedure for experienced urologists, with excellent safety records and predictable outcomes.

The reliability factor represented perhaps the most significant advantage of implant surgery for my situation.

Unlike pills that worked sometimes, injections that required planning and caused discomfort, or vacuum devices that felt unnatural, implants would provide consistent results every time they were activated.

This reliability would eliminate the performance anxiety that plagued other treatment approaches, allowing me to approach intimate situations with confidence rather than apprehension.

Implants would also restore spontaneity to sexual encounters in ways that other treatments could not match. While activation would take thirty to sixty seconds, this brief process could easily become part of foreplay, maintaining the natural flow of intimate encounters.

There would be no waiting for medications to take effect, no interruption for injection procedures, and no need to plan sexual activity hours in advance.

The longevity of implants offered another significant advantage. While pills required ongoing prescriptions and injections needed regular medication refills, implants typically function reliably for fifteen to twenty years or more. This longevity would make them cost-effective compared to ongoing medication expenses, particularly important for me facing potentially decades of treatment costs.

Making My Transition Decision

The decision to pursue implant surgery required careful consideration of multiple factors beyond simple treatment effectiveness. My age, overall health, relationship status, and personal preferences all influenced whether implant surgery represented the right choice for my situation.

Now in my 70's, I was young enough that longevity mattered significantly.

An implant lasting 15-20 years would carry me well into my eighties with reliable function. My overall health was good despite the cardiovascular issues contributing to my ED, making me a good surgical candidate.

My relationship with my girlfriend had been tested by years of erectile dysfunction and failed treatments.

We'd both struggled through disappointing pills, uncomfortable injections, and awkward vacuum devices. She was eager for a reliable solution that would allow us to rebuild our intimacy without the constant anxiety about whether treatments would work.

I traveled frequently and had a demanding schedule that made managing medications or injection supplies logistically challenging. The convenience of an implant over the logistics of ongoing treatments was appealing.

Financial factors influenced my decision as well. Over the device's lifespan, the cost-per-use would be minimal compared to pills or injections.

The psychological readiness for surgery took time to develop.

I'd needed months to process the idea of surgical treatment and mechanical assistance for sexual function.

But after failing with multiple conservative approaches, I felt eager to pursue the most effective available treatment rather than continuing to struggle with unreliable alternatives.

Preparing for Advanced Treatment

Once I'd decided to pursue penile implant surgery, several preparatory steps helped improve my confidence in the process. Education represented the most important preparation, involving thorough understanding of the different implant types, surgical procedures, recovery expectations, and long-term results.

I spent weeks researching qualified specialists who performed implant procedures, and this is presented in more detail in the next two chapters.

I wanted a urologist who understood sexual medicine and had performed a significant number of implant procedures who I knew would offer the best outcomes and lowest complication rates.

A New Beginning, Not an Ending

The failure of pills, injections, vacuum devices, and the inadequacy of speculative treatments for me had felt like the end of my sexual life, but it became an opportunity to discover a treatment that worked better and more reliably than pills ever could.

Modern medicine offered sophisticated solutions for men willing to explore beyond first-line treatments, and the success rates for implants far exceeded what basic medications could provide.

Understanding my options helped transform feelings of hopelessness into realistic optimism about restored sexual function. The journey from pill failure through second-line treatments to surgical solutions required courage and commitment, but thousands of men had walked this path successfully. Their experiences demonstrated that effective solutions existed for virtually every man willing to pursue appropriate treatment.

The decision to move beyond failed conservative therapy represented a choice to stop accepting diminished quality of life and start pursuing the sexual health I deserved. It was a decision to trust modern medical technology and invest in my long-term happiness and relationship satisfaction.

My journey beyond pill failure began with recognizing that better options existed and finding the courage to pursue them.

After years of uncertainty and disappointment, I was finally ready to choose reliability over hope, proven solutions over experimental possibilities.

Later we will explore how I chose the right surgeon for my implant procedure—a decision that proved just as crucial as selecting the right device.

The surgeon you choose will guide you through this process and perform the procedure that could transform your life, making this selection one of the most important decisions in your entire treatment journey.

For supplementary materials, updates, and additional resources mentioned throughout this book, visit:

www.jayrichard.com

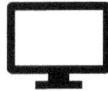

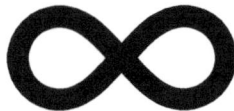

"The best time to plant

a tree was 20 years ago.

The second best time is now."

— Chinese Proverb

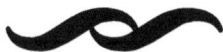

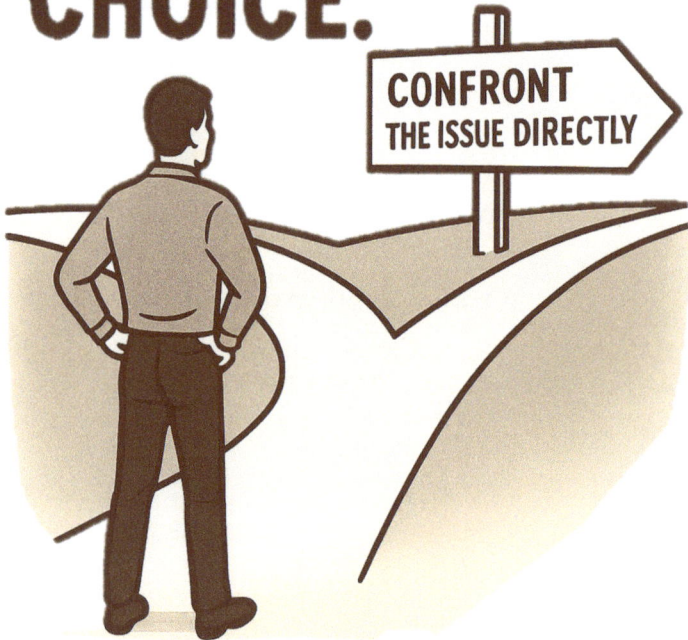

YOU HAVE A CHOICE.

CONFRONT THE ISSUE DIRECTLY

and explore all treatment options.

Know that you CAN reclaim your overall sexual health and well-being.

Chapter 4: Making The Implant Decision
Types, Technology, and Choices

Standing in Dr. Fig's waiting room, clutching a folder full of printed research articles, I felt the weight of the decision before me. The magazines on the coffee table, *Golf Digest, Sports Illustrated,* seemed almost mockingly normal compared to what I was contemplating: permanently replacing a fundamental part of my body's function with a mechanical device.

I'd spent weeks diving deep into medical journals, patient forums, pertinent You Tubes, and manufacturer websites, trying to understand not just the technical differences between implant types, but what choosing each path would actually mean for my daily life.

The statistics I'd found were encouraging—the high satisfaction rates we discussed earlier were backed up by recent research from the American Urological Association.

But statistics only tell part of the story.

What I really needed to understand was this: How would an implant affect not just my sex life, but my confidence in the locker room, my comfort wearing certain clothes, my ability to be spontaneous with my partner?

These were the questions that kept me awake at night, and the answers would determine which direction my life would take.

The Reality of What I Was Choosing

When Dr. Fig called me back to his office, I was ready with a list of detailed questions. I knew where I was going but just wanted to confirm my choice.

He was brutally honest about what would happen undergoing surgery. It became clear that my natural erection mechanism would be gone forever. Most important, that I would not have an enhancement of size, but a replacement of what I had.

Because of the homework I had done, this was not new. It was just confirmation of what I had learned in my study of implants.

When I went home, I sat in my garage for an hour, just thinking and contemplating this decision.

But as the reality settled in, I began to see that for what I wanted out of life, there was only one decision here.

For the past few years, my "natural" function had been anything but natural.

Pills had worked sometimes. Injections were a nightmare of timing and unpredictability.

I was already living with artificial solutions, and the implant would now be the reliable solution I was looking for.

In reality, I was replacing something that was broken with something that was working consistently. A no-brainer for sure!

That's exactly how I began to frame it in my mind.

Instead of mourning the loss of unpredictable natural function, I started imagining what it would feel like to have complete control over my erections for the first time in years.

Navigating the Implant Options

I already knew from my research that there were three types of implants. I wasn't interested in two of the options, the semi-rigid or two-piece systems. Though they might be great for some men, I already knew what I wanted.

The Three-Piece System

This was the one I knew would be perfect for me!

I'd watched countless YouTube videos of the surgery and seen the results in men whose lives had been completely transformed. I believed it was a surgery I could handle.

The doctor would place a separate reservoir in my pelvic area behind the abdominal muscle to hold the fluid necessary for erections and deflation.

Operating the scrotal bulb was straightforward. Just 10-15 pumps of the scrotal bulb to inflate, and when I wanted to deflate, I'd press the release button while gently squeezing the base of my penis. For me, that was easy to understand and operate.

(Note: if you don't have good hand dexterity, you might want to check out the other two options I mentioned above to see if they'd work better for you.)

Most importantly, my research showed that three-piece recipients reported the highest satisfaction scores across every category: erection firmness, natural appearance, partner satisfaction, and overall quality of life improvement.

This was exactly what I wanted!

The Technology That Made It Possible

Part of what gave me confidence was understanding just how sophisticated these devices had become. My research had shown me that modern implants incorporate decades of engineering refinement and materials science advances.

The cylinders themselves were marvels of biomedical engineering, constructed from materials that could expand and contract thousands of times without degrading.

The Engineering Marvel That Will be Inside You

Understanding exactly how my implant was going to work mechanically helped me appreciate the incredible engineering that would soon be living inside my body.

Let me walk you through what would happen when I activated my own three-piece system.

The reservoir behind my abdominal muscle would hold about 100-120ml of sterile saline solution---roughly the amount in a small bottle of contact lens solution. When I squeeze the pump in my scrotum, I'm essentially operating a one-way valve system that forces this fluid through narrow tubing into the cylinders in my penis.

Each cylinder contains an intricate balloon-like structure that can expand both in length and girth as fluid enters. The engineering challenge was enormous: create something that could inflate thousands of times without failing, remain completely bio-compatible, resist infection, and feel as natural as possible.

The pump mechanism itself is a marvel of miniaturization.

It contains multiple one-way valves, a release mechanism, and connection points for the tubing, all in a device smaller than a large grape. When I press the deflation button, I'm opening a valve that allows fluid to return to the reservoir while I gently squeeze the base of my penis to also help move the fluid back to the reservoir.

Does this fascinate you like it did me?

The internal components use proprietary materials designed to last decades while maintaining flexibility and reliability.

What struck me most was learning that each implant is essentially custom fitted during surgery.

Your urologist will measure each anatomy precisely and then select a cylinder length and reservoir capacity specifically for your body.

This is not a one-size-fits-all device-it's personalized medical technology. The fact that this sophisticated hydraulic system would live in a body and operate reliably for 15-20 years seemed almost miraculous.

Modern biomedical engineering had created something that could restore not just function, but confidence and quality of life.

Matching the Decision to My Life

As I worked through the decision over the following days, I realized I needed to be very honest about my lifestyle and priorities.

Being single and still quite active in my seventies, I found myself in plenty of situations where keeping things private was important – work, travel, gym visits, beach trips, you know the drill.

The three-piece system's superior concealment wasn't just cosmetic for me; it was essential for maintaining the normalcy I craved.

My relationship status also influenced the decision. My girlfriend and I had been together for several years, and our sex life had suffered significantly during my struggle with ED. We both wanted the best possible restoration of function, and the three-piece met both our goals.

I also considered my manual dexterity. Research showed that some men with arthritis or neurological conditions might struggle with pump operation, but in my 70's with no hand problems, this wasn't a concern. If anything, having something to actively control appealed to me, it would make me feel like a participant in the process rather than a passive recipient of mechanical function.

Setting Realistic Expectations

I knew that the implant would give me reliable, firm erections suitable for intercourse. It would eliminate performance anxiety and allow for spontaneous sexual activity (after the brief inflation process).

Another thing that I learned was that it wouldn't increase my sexual desire—that had to come from within me. It wouldn't enhance sensation, though most men found sensation remained perfectly adequate.

And it wouldn't increase my size, though improved firmness often created the appearance of increased girth.

What struck me most from my research was learning that the device wouldn't restore spontaneous erections.

With a three-piece system, I'd need to inflate before sexual activity. This seemed like a limitation initially, but as I thought about it, I realized it might be an advantage.

How many times had I struggled with natural erections that came and went unpredictably during intimacy? Having complete control over timing seemed like an improvement, not a compromise.

The Decision Moment

After weeks of research and reflection, I found myself calling Dr. Fig's office to schedule surgery. I had to ask myself: was I sure? Here is how I answered that question. I was sure that years of unpredictable function had affected my confidence, my relationship, and my quality of life more than I'd initially admitted. I was sure that conservative treatments had reached their limits for me. I was sure that the 95% satisfaction rate I'd read about meant something, and that the technology had advanced to the point where complications were rare. Most importantly, I was sure that I was ready to stop accepting diminished sexual function as my new normal. The path forward was clear. I wasn't just choosing a medical device—I was choosing to reclaim control over an essential aspect of my life. The research, the consultation, and the soul-searching had all led to this moment. Now it was time to move from decision to action.

In the next chapter, I'll share how I selected Dr. Fig as my surgeon—a decision that proved just as crucial as selecting the right device.

The surgeon you choose will guide you through this process and perform the procedure that could transform your life, making this selection one of the most important decisions in your entire treatment journey.

∞

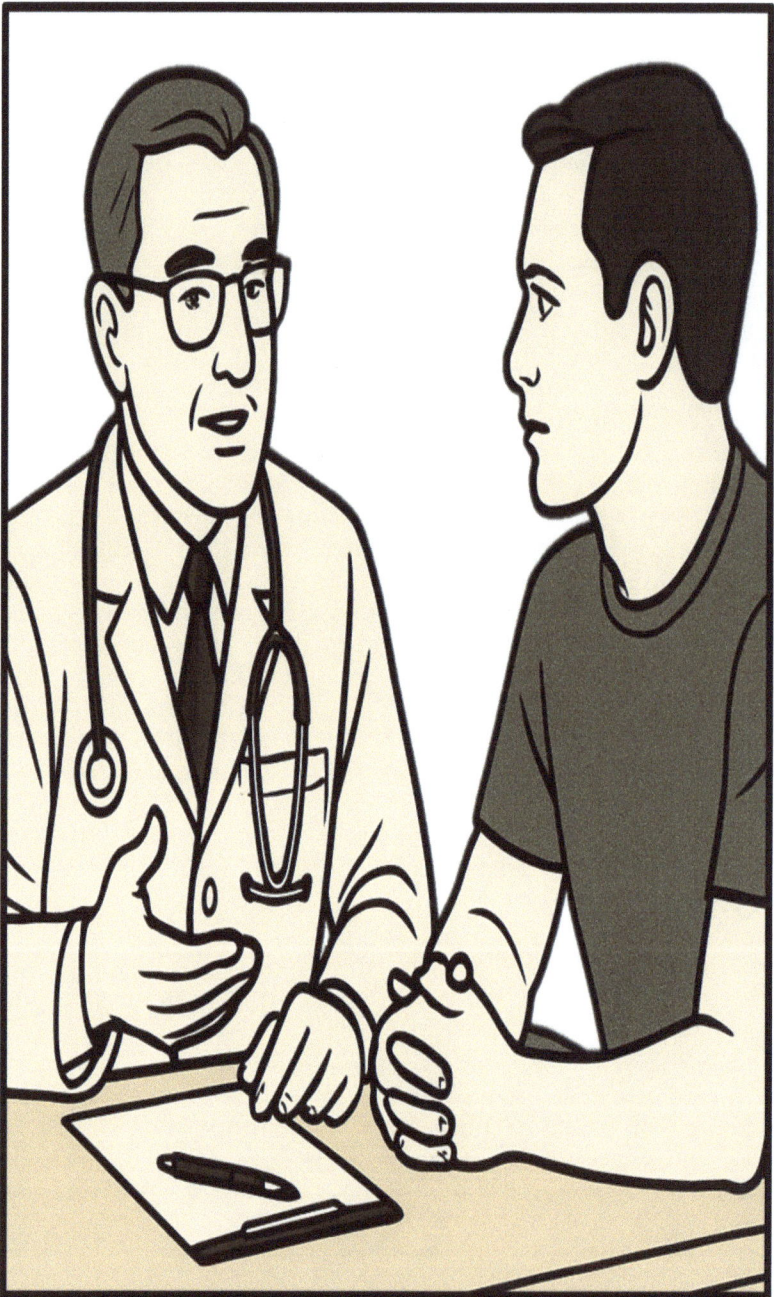

Chapter 5: Choosing Your Surgeon
The Most Critical Decision

Your surgeon choice will determine your outcome for the next 15-20 years.

Beyond avoiding complications, experienced surgeons deliver better results. They understand sizing, positioning, and the nuances that make an implant feel natural rather than mechanical.

Finding the Right Specialist

Most urologists aren't implant specialists. They excel at treating kidney stones, prostate issues, and bladder problems, but penile implants might represent 1-2 procedures monthly at best.

I focused my search on urologists specializing in sexual medicine, doctors with fellowship training who dedicate a significant part of their practice to ED treatment and that were also Board Certified.

Here's some of the organizations where I found them:

Professional Organizations: The American Urological Association directory and Sexual Medicine Society of North America provided sub-specialty searches.

Academic Medical Centers: University hospitals often have sexual medicine specialists who combine practice with research, maintaining higher standards.

Patient Networks: Online forums and previous patients offered valuable insights, though I verified everything independently.

Medical Referrals: My primary care doctor knew which local urologists truly specialized versus those who occasionally performed implants. I consulted with four surgeons. Each taught me what to look for and avoid. One rushed through our appointment in fifteen minutes and couldn't provide specific complication rates. Another was honest about limited experience-20 procedures in two years, but that wasn't sufficient for my comfort. A third was technically qualified but dismissive when I asked about recovery expectations. Since I had been Dr. Fig's patient for many years, he was always my front runner! I felt he met all of what I was looking for but still wanted to go through all the questions below to be sure he was the surgeon I wanted.

The Right Questions
Through trial and error, I developed essential questions that revealed each surgeon's true qualifications:

"How many implants do you perform annually?"
I wanted a doctor that had done a lot. A Doctor that knew what they were doing-I did not want to be a guinea pig.

"What are your infection and complication rates?"
I wanted to see an infection rate under 1%, revision rate around 3% (mostly mechanical issues years later, not surgical complications).

"Which brands do you use and why?"
Quality surgeons use multiple brands and select based on patient anatomy and needs. How did they go about this?

"What's your follow-up process?"
I wanted comprehensive care: scheduled check-ups, 24/7 emergency availability, and ongoing support.

"Can I speak with previous patients?"
References from volunteers willing to share their experiences.

Learning from Others' Mistakes
During research, I heard troubling stories from men who chose their surgeons poorly. One selected a surgeon based solely on insurance coverage, the doctor had minimal implant experience and caused complications requiring multiple revision surgeries.

Another chose the cheapest option and ended up paying twice as much after his implant failed prematurely and required replacement by a specialist.

These weren't isolated incidents. They reinforced that cutting corners on surgeon selection creates far greater problems later.

Why Dr. Fig?

Dr. Fig distinguished himself immediately. Our first consultation lasted over an hour, not from inefficiency, but because he understood this decision's importance.

He addressed the surgery's impact on my entire life, not just the mechanical aspects. His technical answers demonstrated deep expertise from hundreds of procedures. When discussing complications, he was honest about risks and his approach to managing problems.

Most convincingly, every previous patient I spoke with praised his preparation, availability, and results that exceeded expectations.

The Decision

Choosing Dr. Fig was straightforward. He had the experience, outcomes, communication skills, and patient care philosophy I required. Men who choose surgeons based on experience and outcomes rather than convenience or cost consistently report satisfaction with their results. Those who don't often face sub-optimal outcomes or revision surgeries.

Your Path Forward

Invest time in finding a sexual medicine specialist performing many implants yearly. Ask detailed questions about outcomes and complications. Speak with previous patients. Trust your instincts about whether your surgeon understands this procedure's life-changing importance. The extra research time and potential additional cost of choosing the right surgeon could prevent years of problems and thousands in revision surgery expenses. You deserve a surgeon who recognizes they're not just installing a medical device, they're helping restore your confidence, relationships, and quality of life.

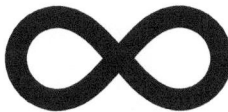

∞

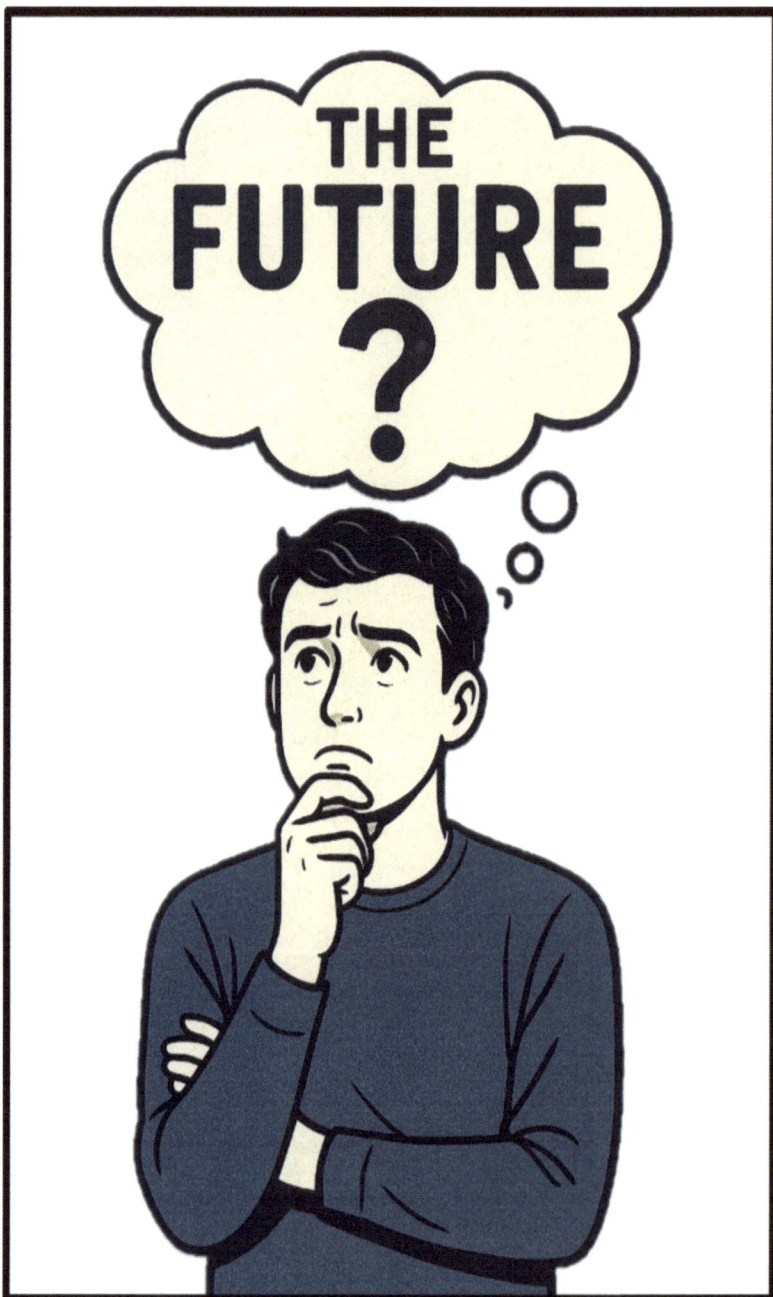

Chapter 6: My Surgery Experience
From Preparation to Recovery

The weeks leading up to my penile implant surgery felt like the longest countdown of my life.

I'd wake up each morning and think, "Twenty-three more days," then "Fifteen more days," then "Holy crap, it's tomorrow."

I was excited, finally doing something definitive about my erectile dysfunction, but I was also terrified. What if something went wrong? What would the pain be like? How long before I'd feel normal again?

Looking back, I realize most of my fear came from not knowing what to expect. My mind filled in the blanks with worst-case scenarios.

That's why I'm writing this chapter to give you the honest, detailed account I desperately wanted but couldn't find anywhere.

Not medical textbook stuff, but what it's really like from someone who's been through it (**remember I am not a doctor, just a guy like you**).

Getting My Body Ready (And My Mind)

About three weeks before surgery, Dr. Fig's office called with a list of things I needed to do. Honestly, it felt overwhelming at first. Blood tests, medication changes, lifestyle adjustments, I thought, "Am I having surgery or training for the Olympics?" The blood work alone required several appointments. They tested everything—my blood count, kidney function, any heart issues, and whether I had any infections lurking around. I appreciated having something to focus on besides my anxiety. The strangest part of preparation was the shower routine. For two days before surgery, I had to shower with this special antibacterial soap called Hibiclens. The stuff smells like a hospital and turns your skin slightly orange. I felt ridiculous scrubbing my entire torso for five minutes like I was prepping for heart surgery, but Dr. Fig assured me it significantly reduces infection risk. My girlfriend joked that I looked like I'd been dunked in iodine.

Preparing for Life After Surgery

While I was getting my body ready, we were also preparing my house for what I thought would be the most uncomfortable week of my recovery.

My biggest decision was where I'd sleep. My bed is high, and I had been warned that getting in and out might be challenging. Luckily, I had a recliner in a spare bedroom, which turned out to be a lifesaver.

For the first four nights, that chair was my home base. I could adjust the position when the swelling got uncomfortable, and I didn't have to worry about rolling onto my surgical site.

My girlfriend went into full preparation mode, stocking up on supplies like we were expecting a blizzard.

Several bags of frozen peas (better than ice packs because they conform to your body), extra-loose sweatpants, slip-on shoes, and enough stool softeners to supply a small pharmacy. I had been advised that pain medications cause constipation, and straining is the last thing you want to do as it could do harm to the device.

The transportation arrangements felt a bit embarrassing. I'm used to being independent, but suddenly I needed to arrange rides like a teenager.

My girlfriend would drive me to the surgery center and back, but we also set up backup plans with friends for follow-up appointments. Looking back, having those plans in place reduced my stress significantly.

The Big Day: 5:30 AM and Rising Panic

Surgery day started ridiculously early.

My procedure was scheduled for 8:00AM, but we had to arrive at 6:00AM, which meant leaving the house at 5:30AM, which meant that horrible antibacterial shower at 5:00AM.

Standing in our bathroom at dawn, washing with that medicinal-smelling soap while my hands trembled slightly, the reality hit me hard: this was happening.

The drive to the hospital was quiet.

My girlfriend kept asking if I was okay, and I kept saying yes, but honestly, I was cycling between excitement and terror every few minutes.

What if I was making a mistake?

What if the recovery was worse than expected?

What if the implant didn't work?

The hospital felt like a cross between a medical office and a hotel lobby—nice but clearly designed to keep you calm.

After checking in and handling the insurance paperwork (tip: look over everything twice because you'll probably forget something), they called my name surprisingly quickly.

Changing into that hospital gown was the point of no return. The nurses were incredibly kind, which helped more than I expected.

They explained every step: "Now we're putting in your IV," "This is just to monitor your heart rate," "The anesthesiologist will be right in." Having someone narrate what was happening kept my mind from racing ahead to things I couldn't control.

When Dr. Fig stopped by for one final check-in, I almost asked him to postpone everything. Not because I'd changed my mind, but because suddenly it felt too real, too immediate.

"Any last questions?" he asked.

I had a million, but they all boiled down to, "Will this work?" and "Will I be okay?"

He must have seen the look on my face because he spent an extra few minutes' reassuring me that this was routine for him and that my case was straightforward.

That's what I needed to hear.

I was ready for surgery!

Waking Up: Not As Bad as I'd Imagined

The next thing I remember was a nurse saying my name and asking how I felt.

For a moment, I couldn't remember where I was or why I was there.

Then it all came flooding back, and my first instinct was to check everything was still attached and working.

The nurse smiled and said, "Everything went perfectly. Don't try to look just yet—you're pretty swollen."

She wasn't kidding.

When I finally worked up the courage to peek under the blanket, I was shocked.

My penis and scrotum were easily twice their normal size and colored like I'd been in a boxing match.

The nurse saw my expression and quickly said, "That's completely normal. It looks much worse than it feels."

She was right, it looked horrifying but felt more like a deep, dull ache than sharp pain.

There was a catheter, which was weird but not painful, and a small drain coming out of my stomach with a little bulb attached to collect fluid. "That'll come out in a few days," the nurse explained. The whole setup looked like something from a sci-fi movie, but knowing it was temporary helped.

Dr. Fig visited while I was in recovery and seemed genuinely pleased.

"Everything went exactly as planned," he said.

"The implant fit perfectly, all the connections are solid, and there were no complications."

Hearing those words was like someone lifting a weight off my chest.

All those weeks of worry, and the actual surgery had gone smoothly.

I knew then that I was going to get my sexual life back!

The First Week: A Day-by-Day Reality Check

Day One:

Getting home was an adventure. Every bump in the road felt magnified, and getting from the car to the house required strategy.

Once I was settled in the recliner with ice packs and pain medication, things became manageable.

The discomfort was there—like someone had kicked me in the groin—but it wasn't the agony I'd feared. Trust me, I had built many "dragons" in my mind, so it was a real relief when none showed up. (Dragons are all the bad things you can imagine, fears that never happen, but you think they could).

Day Two:

The catheter came out this morning, which was both a relief and a new challenge.

My first attempt at urination was an exercise in humility.

The direction was unpredictable, the flow was weak, and it took forever.

It was a little messy.

My girlfriend then wisely suggested sitting down for the next few tries, which saved us both some cleanup time.

Day Three:

This was probably my lowest day emotionally. The swelling seemed worse, I was getting tired of being immobilized, and the reality of having hardware inside my body felt strange. I called Dr. Fig's office with several different concerns, and the nurse patiently addressed each one.

"This is all normal," she kept saying, and hearing that from a professional helped more than I expected.

Day Four:

The drain came out today—just a quick tug that was uncomfortable for about two seconds, then immediate relief at not having that tube attached anymore.

The swelling was starting to go down, and I could see hints of my normal anatomy returning.

Day Five:

First real shower since surgery. It felt amazing to wash properly, though I was extremely gentle around all the surgical sites. The bruising was changing colors—from deep purple to yellow green—which my surgeon had warned me would happen as things healed.

Days Six and Seven:

Each day brought noticeable improvement. I could move around more easily, sleep better, and the pain was manageable with just Tylenol.

I even felt human enough to get annoyed at daytime TV, which my girlfriend said was a good sign.

Week Two: Turning the Corner

By the start of week two, I felt like a different person. The dramatic swelling had subsided enough that I could see my actual anatomy again, though everything was still larger and more colorful than normal. I could walk normally, sleep in our bed, and concentrate on things other than my recovery. The psychological adjustment was harder than the physical healing. Every time I used the bathroom or showered, I was reminded of the hardware inside me. It wasn't painful or problematic—just different. I found myself wondering if it would ever feel completely natural or if I'd always be aware of it.

My two-week follow-up appointment was reassuring. Dr. Fig examined everything, pronounced my healing "excellent," and cleared me to drive. That small bit of independence felt huge.

Weeks Three and Four: Patience, Patience, Patience

Week three brought an unexpected challenge that no one had warned me about: the psychological ups and downs of recovery hit me like a freight train. Physically, I was doing great. The swelling was almost gone, pain was minimal, and I could resume most normal activities. But mentally? I was all over the place. Monday, I felt euphoric. I could see my normal anatomy returning, the incision was healing beautifully, and I was convinced I'd made the best decision of my life. I started planning romantic getaways and feeling like a new man.

Wednesday brought crushing doubt. Looking at my penis, I became convinced it looked different---smaller, somehow wrong. I spent an hour Googling "penile implant regret" and reading horror stories online. By afternoon, I was questioning whether I'd made a terrible mistake. Friday brought anger. I was furious that I had to go through all of this at all.

Why couldn't the pills have kept working? Why couldn't my body just function normally? I snapped at my girlfriend over something trivial and spent the evening apologizing.

This emotional whiplash continued for several days. One moment I felt grateful and optimistic, the next I felt scared and regretful. The worst part was feeling like I couldn't talk about it---who wants to hear about your penis surgery emotions?

Dr. Fig's nurse helped save my sanity. When I called with my concerns, she said, "This is completely normal. You've had surgery on one of the most psychologically significant parts of your body. Your emotions are going to be all over the place for a few weeks. "She was right. The emotional volatility gradually settled as I approached my one-month mark. Looking back, I realize this was part of processing the magnitude of what I had done. I wasn't just healing from surgery---I was mentally adjusting to the reality that my sexual function would never be "natural" again.

If you experience something like this emotional roller coaster, know it's normal and temporary. Most importantly, give yourself time to process this major life change. I needed to keep remembering that this phase was all about waiting for clearance to use my new equipment. When I got down to it, I was feeling mostly normal, could work from home, drive myself places, even take longer walks, but the big question remained: when could I test everything out? "Not yet," Dr. Fig stated. "I know you're eager, but we need complete healing before you put any stress on the surgical sites." It was frustrating but made sense. I'd waited years with ED; I could wait a few more weeks to do things right. The anticipation was building, though.

I could feel the device inside me, could even locate the pump in my scrotum, but I wasn't allowed to operate it yet. It was like having a sports car in the garage with no keys.

Week Four: The Training Day

The day finally arrived—Dr. Fig was going to teach me how to use my implant. I was nervous and excited in equal measure. What if I couldn't figure it out? What if it didn't work? What if it hurt?

"First, let's just find the pump," he said, palpating my scrotum. "Right there-feel that bulb-like structure? That's your control center." Finding it was easier than I expected; it felt like a small, soft walnut nestled in my scrotum. The first inflation was surreal. He guided my fingers to squeeze the pump in a specific rhythm, and suddenly my penis began growing longer and harder. It wasn't painful, just... weird. Like watching magic happen to my own body. "Perfect," he said. "Now let's deflate it. "The deflation process involved finding a different spot on the pump and pressing firmly. It took several tries to get the technique right, but gradually, my penis returned to its flaccid state. "Practice makes perfect," he said. "But don't overdo it, a few times a day at most for the first week."

Eight Weeks: Finally, Back in Business

Dr. Fig cleared me for sexual activity, and that night my girlfriend and I were both nervous. Would it work? Would it feel normal? Would she be able to tell the difference?

Using the pump privately before we attempted anything was smart. I practiced inflating and deflating until I felt confident in my technique. The erection it produced was firm and reliable, harder than anything I'd experienced in years.

The moment of truth arrived. For the first time in years, I approached intimacy without anxiety or uncertainty.

The implant performed flawlessly: reliable, firm, and lasting as long as needed. My partner's satisfaction was obvious, and for the first time in years, I felt like a complete lover again.

I WAS BACK! Hearing my partner say: *"Oh my God, that was fantastic"* validated every moment of discomfort during my recovery. My new ability to achieve an erection on demand, maintain it for as long as desired, and focus entirely on pleasure rather than performance anxiety was transformative.

Looking Back: Worth Every Day of Recovery

Writing this many months later, I can honestly say the surgery and recovery were far less terrible than I'd imagined. Yes, the first week was uncomfortable. Yes, waiting for clearance was frustrating. But compared to years of ED anxiety and failed attempts at intimacy, a few weeks of recovery was nothing.

The hardest part wasn't the physical discomfort, it was the psychological adjustment to having a medical device inside my body. Even now, I'm occasionally aware of it, but it's become as normal as any other part of my anatomy.

If you're facing this surgery, here's what I wish someone had told me: trust the process, follow the instructions, and be patient with yourself. Your body knows how to heal, your surgeon knows what they're doing, and this temporary discomfort is an investment in years of restored confidence and intimacy.

The fear of the unknown is always worse than the reality. Now that I'm on the other side, I wish I'd done this years sooner.

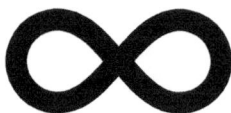

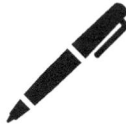

"Courage is not the absence of fear,
but action in spite of it."

— Mark Twain

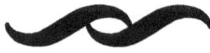

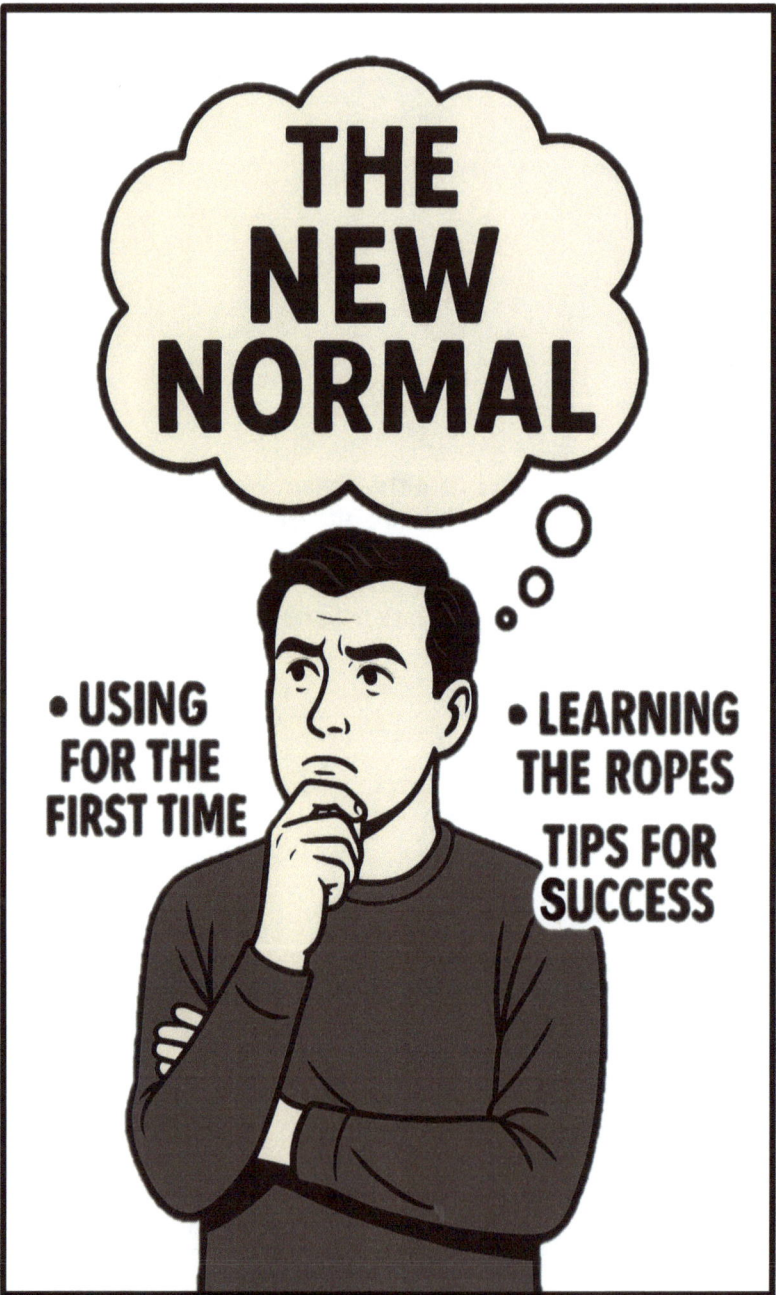

Chapter 7: Life After Surgery
The New Normal

Many months after my penile implant surgery, I can write words I never thought I'd be able to say: **my sex life is better now than it was before ED entered my life**. The reliability, confidence, and freedom from anxiety that my implant provides have transformed not just my sexual experiences, but my entire outlook on relationships and intimacy. This chapter explores what life is really like after successful implant surgery—the good, the challenging, and everything in between.

Physical Changes and Daily Reality

What You'll Actually Experience
The daily awareness of having an implant becomes part of your new normal. You'll feel the implant through movement and positioning, and the cylinders and pump create new physical awareness that requires an adjustment period of several months to feel completely natural. However, this gradual adaptation means that each week feels more normal than the last. When deflated, your flaccid appearance may look slightly different, though this is typically unnoticeable to others. When inflated, the erection is often firmer than natural erections were, providing consistent performance. It's important to understand that the implant restores your natural size rather than enhancing it.

Learning the Mechanics
The inflation process requires ten to fifteen pumps for full erection and takes thirty to sixty seconds to complete. Deflation involves pressing the release valve while gently squeezing the penis base. Daily practice helps maintain familiarity, and understanding normal variations in device response becomes important for troubleshooting.
Practical advantages include inflating when desired without waiting for medication to work, maintaining an erection as long as needed, and complete undetectability when properly deflated. Just remember to deflate after sexual activity.

Return to Full Physical Capacity

After my healing period, I returned to all the activities I enjoyed before—contact sports, swimming, heavy lifting, and every form of exercise. My capacity returned to normal after about six to eight weeks. When I travel, I don't need special considerations for airport security, though I always inform healthcare providers about my implant during medical procedures.

Sexual Function: The Complete Picture

What Remains Unchanged

If you could achieve orgasm before surgery, you still can afterward. Ejaculation typically remains unchanged in both volume and sensation. Sexual pleasure and enjoyment remain intact, and your capacity for intimacy and emotional connection stays the same. The implant doesn't affect libido, so attraction and desire continue unchanged.

What's Dramatically Enhanced

Here's where the magic happens. The implant provides reliability that works every single time without fail—I have a one hundred percent success rate because my device works every time I activate it. All positions become possible, extended sessions can occur without time pressure, and multiple rounds are achievable by deflating, resting, and inflating again. Spontaneity returns through quick activation.

What Requires Adjustment

New considerations include mechanical activation and a brief planning element for preparation. Initially, sensations may feel different than natural erections, and partners need time to adapt to the new firmness.

However, these adjustments become second nature within a few months.

The Psychological Transformation

This is where the real life-changing magic happens. The confidence restoration I experienced goes far beyond the bedroom and touches every aspect of life—not just intimate situations, but professional settings, social gatherings, and quiet moments with my partner.

Eliminating Performance Anxiety Forever

No more worrying about erectile failure. No more constant anxiety affecting enjoyment. No more steering clear of intimate situations. The mental freedom this provides is extraordinary, you can focus on pleasure and connection rather than mechanical function.

Restored Self-Image and Relationship Security

I felt a confidence I hadn't experienced in years. This success rippled into other areas of my life, boosting my general self-confidence. Knowing I could satisfy my partner gave me security in our relationship that I'd forgotten was possible.

For the first time in a long time, I felt optimistic about our intimate future together. The emotional changes bring relief from constant worry, gratitude for restored function, and empowerment through taking control of your medical condition. You develop a new outlook that views sex as pleasure rather than a performance test.

Relationship Impact and Partner Response

When I first told my girlfriend I was considering an implant, I was nervous about her reaction. Her initial response was curiosity, and she had questions about function, relief, and was excited that we might have an improved sex life. After surgery, the first few weeks required patience from both of us as we adapted to the mechanical aspects. What surprised me most was how this renewed our overall connection. We experienced intimacy that had been missing for years, and it strengthened our relationship in ways I hadn't expected. Communication became more important than ever. We gave ourselves permission to experiment and discover what worked best together. The key is approaching disclosure with a matter-of-fact attitude, presenting it as a medical solution, and focusing on positive outcomes.

Real-World Performance and Practical Situations
How It Actually Works Day-to-Day

In real-world scenarios, my implant's versatility amazes me. Spontaneous encounters are possible with just thirty to sixty seconds of activation. Planned intimacy allows preparation ahead of time. Travel situations work normally regardless of location, and stress periods don't affect function like they did with natural erections. What often surprises me is that my device frequently outlasts my natural stamina—it performs longer than my physical endurance. This has led to improved technique because I can focus on pleasure rather than maintaining an erection.

Lifestyle Integration

One of my biggest concerns was whether the implant would change my daily routine or make me feel different. I'm happy to report that my work and social life continue exactly as they did before. The implant is completely private—no one knows unless I choose to tell them, and honestly, most of the time I forget it's even there.

Managing Challenges and Expectations

Minor Issues and Solutions

In my early months, I occasionally experienced slight auto-inflation during the day and some difficulty with deflation while learning proper technique. I noticed temporary sensitivity changes that required adjustment. My solutions involved regular practice to improve technique and patience—most issues resolved with time and experience. When I had persistent problems, I didn't hesitate to contact Dr. Fig for guidance.

Measuring Success: Personal and Medical

From a medical perspective, I'm part of the over ninety-five percent of patients who achieved functional erections with high device reliability. I'm also among the over ninety percent who are satisfied with their implants. I absolutely would choose this procedure again. My personal success indicators are clear: restored sexual confidence, improved relationship satisfaction, eliminated performance anxiety, return to normal sexual activities, and overall improvement in life satisfaction. These changes have exceeded my expectations and transformed my quality of life.

Before and After: The Real Comparison
Before Implant Reality

Unreliable erections where you never knew if it would work, constant performance anxiety affecting enjoyment, limited positions, pressure to climax quickly before losing erection, partner frustration, and avoidance of intimate situations.

After Implant Reality

Reliable function that works every single time, eliminated performance worry, full range of sexual activities, extended sessions lasting as long as desired, consistent partner satisfaction, and renewed pursuit of intimate situations.

Special Situations and Disclosure

Navigating New Relationships

Disclosure is a personal choice about timing, often best handled before the first sexual encounter. A matter-of-fact approach works best, focusing on positive function and educating about safety and sensation. Most partners focus on the relationship rather than medical details.

Professional and Social Life

The implant has no impact on job performance, physical demands, or travel requirements. Medical privacy remains protected. Potential positive impacts include increased confidence improving professional demeanor and better focus without distraction from performance concerns.

Long-Term Outlook and Future Planning

Device Longevity and Maintenance

Modern implants typically last fifteen to twenty years. Daily use doesn't significantly impact longevity, and when my device eventually needs service, replacement is possible. Maintenance requirements are minimal—just normal hygiene and regular use to maintain familiarity.

Technology and Replacement Considerations

Device reliability continues improving, surgical techniques are becoming less invasive, materials are more durable, and better technology will be available when replacement becomes needed. Insurance usually covers mechanical failure, and each generation performs better than the last.

Advice for New Implant Recipients

First Month Recommendations
Focus on healing first without rushing into sexual activity. Learn your device by practicing inflation and deflation regularly. Keep your partner involved in the process and manage expectations—full adaptation takes several months.

Long-Term Success Strategies
Use your device regularly to maintain familiarity. Maintain open communication with your partner about your experiences. Schedule annual check-ups with your urologist. Stay informed about advances in implant technology.

Focus on benefits rather than limitations. Avoid common mistakes: overusing initially, neglecting your partner's adjustment needs, skipping follow-ups, and feeling shame instead of accepting this as normal medical treatment.

Words of Encouragement For Those Considering Surgery
From someone who's been through it: the anxiety is worse than the reality.

Recovery represents temporary discomfort for long-term benefit.

Results exceed expectations—most men are thrilled with outcomes, and relationships often improve with better intimacy than before the procedure.

For Those Recently Post-Surgery
Patience is crucial.

Healing takes time, so don't judge results too early.

Each week gets better—gradual improvement is normal.

Remember why you chose this solution and know that support is available through your medical team and online communities.

Final Thoughts: A Life Transformed

Two plus years after surgery, the decision to get a penile implant continues to be one of the best choices I've ever made. The temporary discomfort and adjustment period pale in comparison to the life-changing benefits. Daily reality brings confidence without anxiety, improved relationship quality through better intimacy and communication, and general life improvement with positive effects extending beyond the bedroom.

This represents an investment in quality of life that pays dividends daily.

You deserve to be happy, confident, and sexually fulfilled. The tools exist to make that happen, the choice is yours to use them.

Life after penile implant surgery isn't just about restored sexual function, it's about reclaiming joy, confidence, and the full experience of intimate relationships.

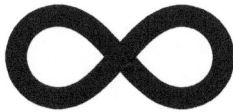

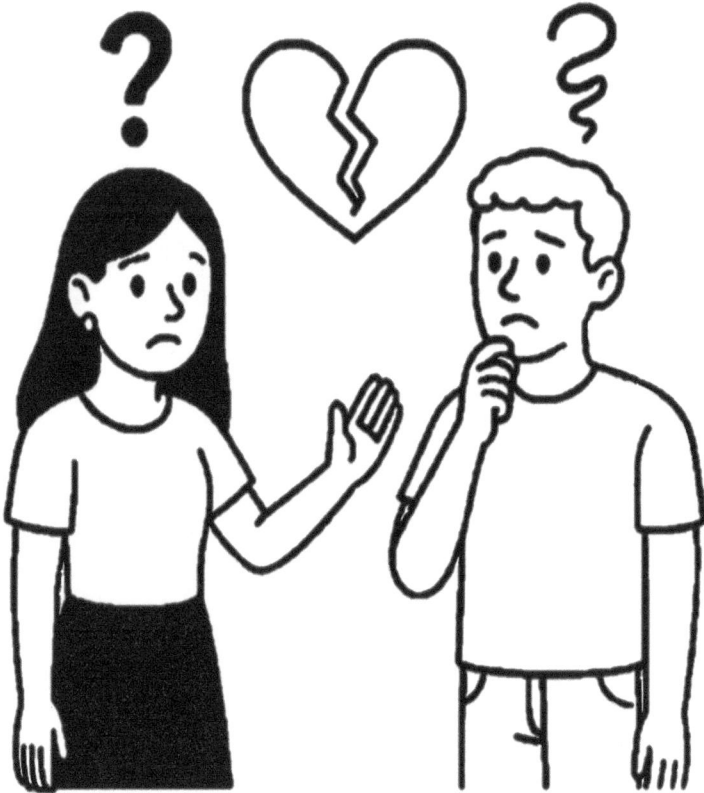

Partner's Thoughts:

- Rejection
- Unattractiveness
- Confused

Chapter 8: For Partners
Navigating This Journey Together

I wrote this chapter specifically for you, the partner of a man dealing with erectile dysfunction. If you're feeling confused, hurt, or somehow responsible for what's happening, I want you to know you're not alone. I've walked this path myself, and I understand how isolating it can feel.

As we established in the opening chapters: **Erectile dysfunction is a medical condition, not a reflection of your attractiveness, your relationship, or anything you've done wrong.**
During my journey with ED, I discovered that partners often become the forgotten participants in this experience, even though you're profoundly affected by both the condition and its treatment. I want you to know that your feelings matter, your concerns are completely valid, and your support can make the difference between treatment success and failure.

Understanding What's Really Happening
Let me explain ED the way I wish someone had explained it to me when I first started dealing with this condition.
I came to understand it as essentially a plumbing problem combined with an electrical issue. The blood vessels that should fill the penis become damaged or blocked, while the nerve signals that should trigger everything become disrupted. What I experienced was this: my brain would send all the right signals, telling my body exactly what I wanted to happen, but my body simply wasn't cooperating anymore. This disconnect between what I desperately wanted and what my body could do created enormous frustration and led me to withdraw emotionally, something you might be witnessing in your own partner.
The hardest lesson I had to accept was that my feelings for my partner hadn't changed. My love and attraction remained completely intact. The disconnect was purely physical, between my mind's desire and my body's ability to respond. I discovered that no amount of mental effort could overcome damaged blood vessels or disrupted nerve signals.

Your Emotional Journey

From what I've observed and experienced, the range of emotions you're feeling is completely normal and shared by millions of partners facing similar situations. I've seen partners feel rejected and question their own appeal, become frustrated that simple solutions don't seem to work, or feel guilty for wanting intimacy when their partner is struggling. I've witnessed the real grief that comes from losing spontaneous intimacy, the fear about what the future holds, and the isolation that develops because ED remains somewhat taboo to discuss openly. I want you to know that all these feelings are valid and deserve acknowledgment rather than being minimized or pushed aside.

Understanding His Experience

I can tell you from personal experience that men dealing with ED face shame and embarrassment at the very core of our being. I tied my masculine identity closely to sexual performance, making ED feel like fundamental failure rather than a medical condition requiring treatment. What I experienced was an anxiety cycle that fed on itself: my worry about performance made the physical problem worse, which created more anxiety, making the next encounter even more likely to fail.

What Your Partner Wants You to Know

After speaking with dozens of partners whose men have navigated ED and implant surgery, I've discovered there are crucial things partners desperately want to communicate but often don't know how. Here's what they wish you understood:

"I miss the intimacy more than the sex."

Partners consistently told me that losing casual physical affection—hand-holding, cuddling, spontaneous kisses— affected them more deeply than the absence of intercourse. When men withdraw physically to avoid sexual expectations, partners feel rejected in ways that extend far beyond the bedroom.

"I blame myself even though I know better."

Despite understanding that ED is medical, partners often wonder if they're still attractive enough, if they caused the problem, or if you would function normally with someone else. This self-doubt can be devastating and requires direct, ongoing reassurance.

"I'm afraid to bring it up because I don't want to pressure you."

Partners want to discuss the situation but fear any conversation will feel like sexual pressure. They need explicit permission to express their feelings and concerns without worrying about making things worse.

"I want to support you, but I don't know how."

Many partners feel helpless watching you struggle. They crave guidance about how to be genuinely supportive during treatment and recovery, rather than accidentally saying or doing the wrong thing.

"I'm grieving too, and I need you to understand that."

Partners experience real loss, the spontaneous intimate life you once shared is gone, even if something better will replace it. This grief needs acknowledgment and space to process together.

"I need to understand what's happening medically."

Partners often want information about ED and treatment options but feel uncomfortable asking. Including them in medical consultations and sharing what you're learning can strengthen your partnership through this process.

"I worry about your mental health more than the physical symptoms."

Partners frequently notice depression, anxiety, and withdrawal that you might not recognize in yourself. They worry about the psychological impact and wonder when to suggest professional help.

"I need reassurance that we have an intimate future together."

Whether through treatment or adaptation, partners need to know that intimacy-in whatever form-remains part of your shared vision for the relationship.

The overwhelming message I heard from every partner was this:

"Please don't shut us out."

Partners want to be part of the solution, not another source of pressure. The silence and withdrawal that often accompany ED can damage relationships more than the condition itself. Your partner chose to be with you through health challenges, let them.

Starting Conversations

One thing that struck me during my medical appointments was how naturally doctors discussed ED. They approached it with complete professionalism, treating it as a common medical condition rather than something shameful. Their matter-of-fact attitude helped me realize I needed to bring that same energy to conversations with my partner. Through trial and error, I learned that timing and setting make all the difference. My first attempt at "the talk" was a disaster, I brought it up right before bed, in our bedroom, after we'd both had a stressful day. She felt ambushed, I felt defensive, and we both ended up more frustrated than before. What worked was choosing moments when we were both relaxed and unhurried. Weekend mornings over coffee became our sweet spot, though quiet evenings after dinner worked too. The key was avoiding any setting that felt sexually charged or pressured.

I also learned not to dive straight into the medical details. Instead, I started broader: "I've been thinking about us lately, and I want to make sure we're both feeling good about our relationship. I love you, and there are some things I'd like us to talk about openly." This approach gave her permission to share what was on her mind too, rather than making it all about my condition. Some of our most important conversations started with her concerns, not mine. The biggest mistake I made early on was trying to solve everything in one conversation. I'd overwhelm her with research, treatment options, timelines, and expectations. What I discovered was that these conversations work better as an ongoing dialogue rather than a single "state of the union" address. Now I try to wrap up these talks by acknowledging that we're building something together: "I'm grateful we can talk about this honestly. There's no pressure or timeline from me, I just want us to stay connected as we figure this out." The goal isn't to have the perfect conversation. It's to start having real conversations instead of dancing around the subject while we both suffer in silence.

How ED Affected My Relationship
I can share what I observed in my own relationship.
The changes began before sexual activity stopped entirely.
I noticed that sexual attempts became less frequent because my anxiety about potential failure made every intimate moment feel risky. I found that romantic situations that once brought us closer began creating tension instead. What I experienced was the loss of casual physical intimacy that bonds couples—I became hyper-vigilant about any contact that might create sexual expectations, so I stopped the hand-holding, quick kisses, and playful touching throughout the day. Perhaps most difficult was the emotional distance I created. I withdrew to protect both of us from disappointment, but I realize now that this protective behavior often created exactly the relationship problems I was trying to prevent.

Providing Support and Maintaining Intimacy
From my journey, I learned that your support could make an enormous difference in both his treatment success and your relationship's survival. What I found most helpful was when my girlfriend maintained physical connection through non-sexual touching: holding my hand while watching TV, giving back rubs without expectation, cuddling while reading, and maintaining affectionate touches throughout our day. I responded well to supportive language like, "I love you exactly as you are" and "This medical condition doesn't change how I feel about you." What made things worse was when I heard phrases that increased pressure, like suggestions to "just relax and it will work." What I discovered is that intimacy extends far beyond sexual activity. We strengthened our emotional bonds through deep conversations, shared activities, and date nights that didn't create sexual pressure. I learned that sexual intimacy could be redefined through oral intimacy, manual stimulation, and thoughtful use of toys. What helped me most was understanding that orgasm wasn't the only goal of our intimate time together.

Treatment Support and Professional Help

When I was considering penile implant surgery, my partner's support significantly influenced both my decision and the procedure's ultimate success. What made the biggest difference was how we learned about the procedure together and discussed our expectations openly. During my recovery, she provided practical support with household tasks, transportation, and monitoring my progress while being incredibly patient with the mood changes that came from pain and medication. We also considered couples counseling when our attempts to communicate about this consistently led to arguments, when we felt disconnected despite our efforts to stay close, and honestly, when we both wondered if our relationship could survive this challenge. What I can tell you from my personal experience is that after successful treatment, our sexual relationship became even better than it had been before ED developed. Accordingly, through this journey, we learned to communicate more openly about everything, not just sex, and we discovered how to focus on overall intimacy rather than just performance.

My Hope for Your Future Together

I want to share what I discovered about the other side of this journey because when you're dealing with ED, it's hard to imagine things getting better. But I've lived it, and I've watched other couples live it too.

What happened in my relationship once we found the right approach surprised me. Beyond restored sexual function and renewed confidence, we became much better at talking about intimate topics, the constant anxiety finally lifted, and spontaneous affection returned to our daily lives.

The deeper changes took time to recognize. We developed communication skills that improved our entire partnership. The emotional intimacy and trust we built facing this challenge together created a foundation stronger than before. I found myself appreciating what we had in ways I never had, and we both gained confidence that we could handle whatever came our way as a team.

Your love and support matter more than you probably realize. When my girlfriend stood with me through this challenge, her willingness to understand, support, and grow with me demonstrated a depth of commitment that was amazing. That commitment, combined with working on our relationship together, restored not just my sexual function but the joy and intimacy that made our relationship truly fulfilling.

What I can promise from my experience is that with the right approach and mutual support, your relationship can become better than it was before ED developed. I believe in your ability to not just overcome this challenge but to emerge stronger, more connected, and more satisfied together than ever before.

What I learned is that your love and support matter more than you probably realize. When my girlfriend stood with me through this challenge, she wasn't just helping me regain sexual health, we were building a stronger, more resilient relationship that could weather any storm.

The truth I want you to hold onto is this: ED was temporary once I got proper treatment, but the strength we built together by facing this challenge could not have been done alone.

My girlfriend's willingness to understand, support, and grow with me demonstrated a depth of commitment and love that was amazing. That commitment, combined with modern medical treatments, restored not just my sexual function but the joy and intimacy that made our relationship truly fulfilling. Looking back on everything we went through; I want you to remember what I've said before: ED is a medical condition that has nothing to do with you personally. Your feelings and concerns are completely valid. Communication forms the foundation for navigating this challenge successfully, and multiple effective treatment options exist with high success rates. Intimacy extends far beyond sexual activity, professional help is available when you need it, and many couples not only overcome ED but build stronger relationships in the process.

What I can promise you from my own experience is that with proper treatment and mutual support, your relationship can become better than it was before ED developed. I've lived this transformation, I've witnessed it in other couples, and I believe in your ability to not just overcome this challenge but to emerge stronger, more connected, and more satisfied together than ever before.

A Message for Partners

Throughout this journey, I've learned and discussed that ED doesn't just affect the man experiencing it—it impacts relationships, partners, and families in profound ways.

While writing this book, I kept thinking about my girlfriend and how she navigated this challenging time with me. Her questions, concerns, fears, and hopes deserved their own dedicated resource. That's why I'm excited to share that I'm completing a companion book specifically written for partners. As noted in this chapter, too often, partners feel left out of the conversation, unsure how to help, what to say, or how to process their own emotions about ED and potential treatments like implant surgery.

Keep Your Eyes Open For The Companion Book:

"When Hope Feels Lost: A Complete Guide to Supporting Him Through Treatment"

A Heartfelt Resource for Partners

This companion book addresses the questions I heard from my partner and others: "How do I support him without making it worse?" "What should I expect during recovery?" "How will this affect our relationship?" "Is it normal for me to feel frustrated, scared, or confused?"

Just as this book provided honest, real-world guidance for men facing intimate health challenges, the partner's guide offers the same authentic perspective for those who love and support them. Because healing and restoration work best when both people in a relationship understand the journey ahead.

If you found value in this book, please share it with the important people in your life. And if your partner could benefit from their own dedicated resource, watch for "When Hope Feels Lost."

Recovery is a team effort. Both of you deserve support, understanding, and hope for the future!

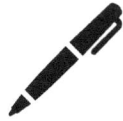

"You are braver than you believe,
stronger than you seem,
and more capable than you imagine."

— A.A. Milne

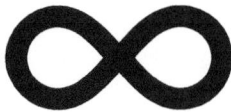

FINANCIALS

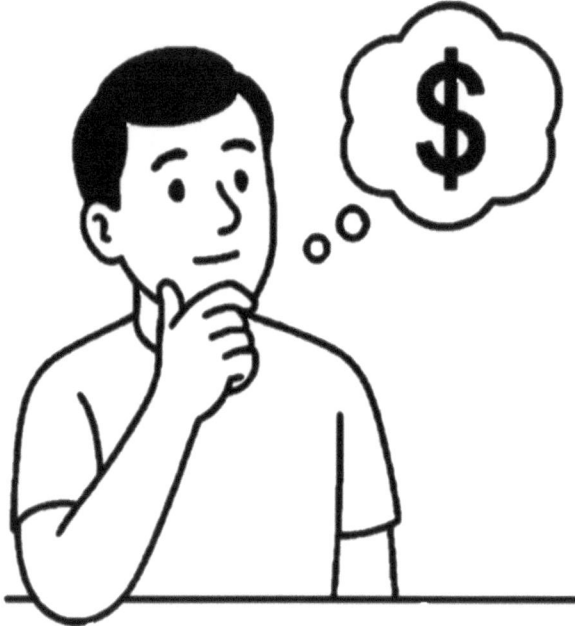

- Cost
- Insurance
- Investment

Chapter 9: Financial Considerations
Cost, Insurance, and Investment

The elephant in the room that no one likes to discuss openly is this simple truth: penile implant surgery can be expensive without insurance. When I first started researching costs, the numbers felt overwhelming. The sticker shock almost derailed my decision entirely, until I began to understand something crucial: this wasn't just a medical expense, it was an investment in the next fifteen to twenty years of my life. I'm sharing my financial journey honestly because money shouldn't be the only factor that prevents you from reclaiming your sexual health, but financial stress shouldn't compromise your recovery either.

This chapter addresses the financial reality head-on, providing honest cost information and practical strategies.

Facing the Real Numbers

When I started getting quotes, penile implant surgery ranged from fifteen thousand to thirty thousand dollars for everything. The wide range shocked me until I understood what drove the differences: geographic location, surgeon experience, implant type, and facility costs. What helped me process these numbers was breaking them down over time. A twenty-thousand-dollar implant lasting fifteen years equals about one hundred eleven dollars per month. When I compared that to the nearly two hundred dollars I was already spending monthly on ED medications that barely worked, the implant ultimately represented significant savings for me. This perspective shift changed everything. Rather than seeing this as a crushing expense, I began viewing it as a strategic investment in my quality of life, relationship, and overall happiness for the next two decades.

Navigating Insurance Coverage

I learned that most insurance plans, including Medicare, cover penile implants when they're deemed medically necessary.

The key word is "necessary," which means you must prove you've tried other treatments first and that ED is significantly impacting your life. Dr. Fig's office handled the pre-authorization process expertly. They submitted detailed documentation of my ED history, records of failed oral medications and injection therapy, lab results, and a letter explaining why an implant was my best option. My insurance company took three weeks to respond, and during that time, I couldn't schedule surgery. When approval finally came, I was covered by Medicare and my supplemental insurance except for my usual deductible and coinsurance. Others have told me they experienced similar coverage levels. I learned that final denials are rare when the medical criteria are clearly met, so if you receive an initial denial, don't give up. Appeals often succeed with additional documentation.

Making It Work Financially
For those facing significant out-of-pocket costs, several strategies can help reduce the financial burden:

Strategic Timing:
If you've already met your annual deductible through other medical expenses, your out-of-pocket cost becomes just your coinsurance. Consider where you are in your plan year when planning surgery.

Cash Payment Discounts:
Many surgical practices offer ten to twenty percent discounts for patients paying the full amount upfront. Always ask about this option.

Smart Financing Options:
Medical credit cards like CareCredit can work if you can pay during their promotional zero-interest period, but the interest rates afterward are brutal. I found a personal loan from my credit union offered much better terms. Shop around carefully.

Health Savings Account Strategy:
For those with high-deductible health plans, maximizing your HSA contribution can significantly reduce your net cost while providing tax advantages. Others have told me this approach turned a major medical expense into a sophisticated tax-planning opportunity.
Consult with a financial adviser to optimize this strategy for your specific situation.

Avoiding Common Financial Mistakes

Don't assume insurance coverage.
Get written pre-authorization before committing to anything. Call your insurance company directly—not just the general customer service line—to understand your exact benefits for this procedure.

Be wary of prices that seem too good to be true.
One surgeon quoted significantly less than others, but when I researched further, I discovered he had limited experience with implants. This isn't the place to bargain hunt on quality.

Read financing agreements carefully.
Some medical credit cards have predatory terms. Taking time to shop around for financing can save you hundreds in interest.

My Planning Process
I approached this systematically by first calling my insurance company to understand my exact benefits. Then I compared all payment options and timed the surgery strategically within my plan year. This planning approach allowed me to focus on the medical and personal factors that mattered most, rather than worrying about money.

I also researched surgeons thoroughly, understanding that experience and expertise were worth paying for. The difference between a successful outcome and complications far outweighed any cost savings from choosing a less experienced surgeon.

Making the Decision
This could be one of your largest medical expenses, but when you honestly evaluate the ongoing costs of ineffective treatments, the impact on your relationship, and the effect on your overall happiness, the investment makes sense. Ask yourself two critical questions: "Can I afford this without compromising essential needs?" and "Can I afford NOT to do this?" When you consider the ongoing medication costs, relationship stress, and personal unhappiness, the answers should become very clear. What convinced me was realizing this investment would affect my quality of life for the next fifteen to twenty years. The restoration of sexual confidence,

improvement in my relationship, and elimination of performance anxiety affected every aspect of my life. I became more confident at work, more present in social situations, and genuinely happier. How do you put a price on that? Looking back, it was one of the best investments I've ever made, not just financially, but in every aspect of my life that mattered. The temporary financial stress was worth the permanent improvement in my quality of life.

The Bottom Line

Don't let financial concerns prevent you from exploring this option, but don't ignore them either. With proper planning, insurance advocacy, and strategic timing, the cost can be manageable. More importantly, when you consider the long-term benefits to your health, relationships, and happiness, this investment in yourself makes perfect financial and personal sense.

The key is approaching this decision with both your heart and your calculator. Your future self will thank you for both the courage to proceed and the wisdom to plan it properly.

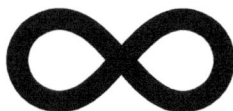

∞

?

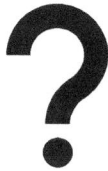

THE QUESTIONS YOU NEED ANSWERED

Knowledge reduces fear.
Understanding builds confidence.
Information empowers decisions.

The following FAQ section addresses the concerns
most men have but are sometimes hesitant to ask.

Your questions matter. Here are the answers.

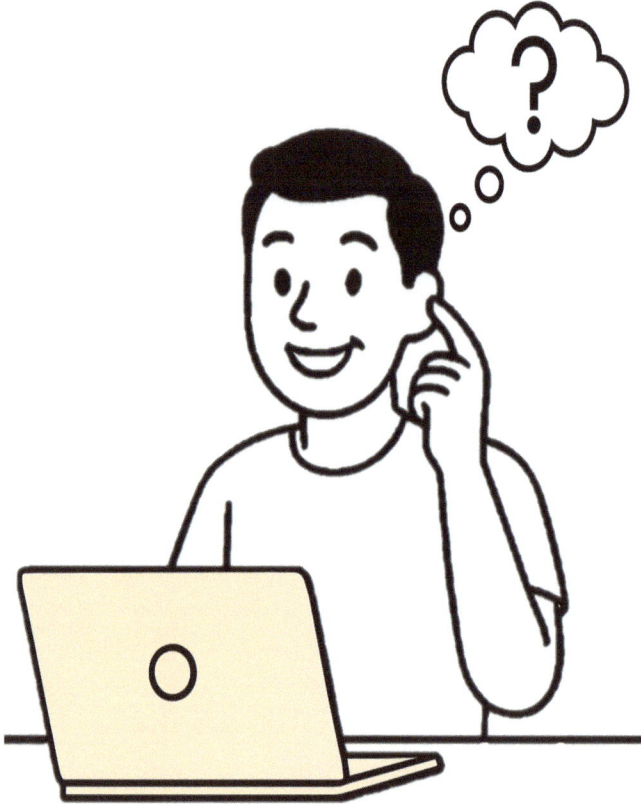

FREQUENTLY
ASKED
QUESTIONS

Chapter 10: Frequently Asked Questions

This section addresses common questions that don't fit neatly into other chapters but are important for understanding penile implants.

Pre-Surgery Questions

Q: How do I know if I'm a good candidate for an implant?

Good candidates typically have diagnosed erectile dysfunction for six months or longer, failed response to pills, injections, or other treatments, realistic expectations about outcomes, good overall health for surgery, and either a stable relationship or clear personal goals. Poor candidates may have untreated psychological causes of ED, unrealistic expectations about size enhancement, active infections or serious medical conditions, or substance abuse problems affecting healing.

Q: Can I get an implant if I've never tried pills or other treatments?

Most surgeons and insurance companies require documentation of failed conservative treatments first. However, in rare cases where pills are contraindicated due to certain heart conditions, implants may be considered as first-line treatment.

Q: What if I have Peyronie's disease (curved penis)?

Penile implants can often correct curvature while restoring erectile function. Many surgeons can address both issues in a single procedure, though severe curvature may require additional surgical techniques.

Q: Can I get an implant if I'm diabetic?

Yes, but diabetes requires special consideration. Blood sugar must be well-controlled before surgery, there's a higher infection risk requiring careful monitoring, healing may take longer, but most diabetic men do very well with implants.

Q: What's the minimum or maximum age for implant surgery?

No strict age limits exist, but considerations vary by age group. Younger men must demonstrate clear medical need and maturity, while for older men, overall health matters more than age. The most common age range is fifty to seventy-five years old.

Surgery and Recovery Questions

Q: Can I choose my implant type, or does the surgeon decide?

This should be a shared decision based on your preferences and lifestyle, surgeon's recommendation based on your anatomy, manual dexterity for pump operation, and cost and insurance considerations.

Q: What happens if I get an erection during surgery?

This cannot happen once the implant is placed, as it replaces your natural erectile mechanism. Any erection during early surgery phases is managed by the surgical team.

Q: How long before I can drive after surgery?

Typically, three to seven days, depending on pain medication use (never drive while taking narcotic pain medications), comfort sitting for extended periods, ability to perform emergency maneuvers, and your surgeon's specific recommendations.

Q: Can I fly after surgery?

Generally safe after one to two weeks, but consider increased swelling risk from pressure changes, comfort sitting for extended periods, access to medical care if complications arise, and your surgeon's clearance for travel.

Q: When can I return to work?

This depends on your job type. Desk jobs typically allow return in three to seven days, physical labor requires four to six weeks, heavy lifting needs six to eight weeks, and driving or traveling jobs usually permit return in one to two weeks.

Q: What about exercise and sports?

The timeline for activity return includes walking, which is immediately encouraged, light exercise after two to three weeks, weightlifting after six to eight weeks, contact sports after eight to twelve weeks, and swimming after incisions are fully healed in two to three weeks.

Functional Questions

Q: Will my partner be able to tell I have an implant?

When properly healed and deflated, the implant is usually undetectable visually, may feel slightly different by touch but not obviously artificial, functions normally during sex with typically high partner satisfaction, and the pump located in the scrotum is not normally touched during intimacy.

Q: Can the implant break during sex?

Modern implants are extremely durable, designed to withstand normal sexual activity with no reported cases of breakage during typical use. You should avoid extreme positions initially while healing, and mechanical failure usually occurs gradually rather than suddenly.

Q: What if I want to have children after the implant?

Implants don't affect fertility. Sperm production remains unchanged, ejaculation stays normal if it was normal before surgery, there's no impact on ability to father children, and fertility testing can be done normally.

Q: Can I still masturbate with an implant?

Yes, this is completely normal. Wait until healing is complete at six to eight weeks, use the pump to inflate as needed, remember to deflate afterward, and understand that sensation may be different initially but normalizes over time.

Q: What about oral sex for my partner?

No restrictions exist once healed. The implant doesn't affect taste or safety, partners cannot be harmed by the device, and it functions normally for all sexual activities.

Lifestyle Questions

Q: Can I go through airport security with an implant?

Yes, no special considerations are needed. Metal detectors cannot detect modern implants, no special documentation is required, there's no need to inform security personnel, and you can travel normally without restrictions.

Q: What about MRI scans?

These are generally safe. Modern implants are MRI-compatible, though you should inform the radiology technician about your implant. The device may cause minor image artifacts but creates no safety concerns with magnetic fields.

Q: Can I get other surgeries after having an implant?

Yes, but inform all healthcare providers about your implant. Urological procedures may require special precautions, abdominal surgeons should know about reservoir location, cardiac procedures have no expected interactions, and general anesthesia creates no additional risks.

Q: What about hot tubs, saunas, and extreme temperatures?

No restrictions apply. Implants are unaffected by temperature changes, normal heat and cold exposure is fine, and there's no risk of malfunction from temperature variations.

Relationship Questions

Q: How do I tell a new partner about my implant?

This is a personal choice but consider timing before intimacy but after trust is established, approach the topic matter-of-factly focusing on positive function, provide education explaining that function is normal though mechanically assisted, and maintain confidence as your attitude will influence their reaction.

Q: What if my partner is uncomfortable with the idea?

Common concerns and appropriate responses include addressing safety concerns by explaining it's completely safe with no risk to partners, acknowledging it may feel slightly different but remains pleasurable, clarifying that ED is medical rather than attraction-related, and considering couples counseling if significant resistance exists.

Q: Can we be spontaneous, or do we always need to plan ahead?

Spontaneity remains possible. Inflation takes thirty to sixty seconds, similar to applying a condom, can become part of foreplay, partners can learn to operate the pump if desired, and this is much more spontaneous than planning around pills.

Complications and Troubleshooting

Q: What if my pump gets stuck or won't work?

Don't panic. Try gentle manipulation first, contact your surgeon's office for guidance, understand that most "stuck" pumps just need proper technique, and know that true mechanical failure is uncommon but repairable.

Q: What if I develop an infection?

Seek immediate medical attention. Early signs include fever, increasing pain, redness, and drainage. Treatment may require antibiotics or device removal. Prevention involves following all post-operative care instructions. Even if device removal is needed, replacement is usually possible.

Q: Can the implant deflate on its own?

Slow deflation can occur. Gradual deflation of a small amount over hours is normal, sudden deflation may indicate a mechanical issue, complete deflation usually indicates a valve problem, and any concerns should prompt contact with your surgeon for evaluation.

Q: What if I'm not satisfied with the results?

Options exist for addressing concerns. Minor issues often resolve with time and experience, sizing concerns may be addressed with revision surgery, mechanical problems can usually be corrected, and while complete dissatisfaction may lead to removal, this is irreversible.

Cost and Practical Questions

Q: Is revision surgery covered by insurance?

Coverage usually applies for mechanical failure. Warranty coverage means the device manufacturer may cover replacement, insurance typically covers medically necessary revisions, patient dissatisfaction may not be covered, and infection-related revisions are usually covered.

Q: What if I lose my job and insurance after surgery?

Plan ahead by considering COBRA to continue coverage temporarily, manufacturer programs that may offer patient assistance, surgeon payment plans that may be available for follow-up care, and emergency care that's always available regardless of insurance status.

Q: Can I get a second opinion after seeing one surgeon?

This is absolutely recommended. Different perspectives mean surgeons may have different approaches, comfort level is important for feeling confident in your choice, most insurance plans cover second opinion consultations, and you should prepare the same questions for consistency.

Q: What if my surgeon retires or moves?

Plan for continuity by ensuring you have copies of medical records, knowing your exact implant model, understanding that most local urologists can provide follow-up care, and knowing that manufacturer support can help locate qualified surgeons.

Technical Questions

Q: How do I know which brand or model is best?

Consider your surgeon's expertise by using what your surgeon knows best, your anatomy as some models fit certain anatomies better, personal preferences regarding ease of use, concealment and firmness, and insurance coverage which may limit brand options.

Q: Can implants be upgraded to newer technology?
Not typically through simple upgrade. Replacement surgery can allow choosing a newer model if replacement is needed, elective upgrades are usually not medically necessary or covered, technology improvements are gradual rather than revolutionary, and current devices are already very advanced and reliable.

Q: What happens to my natural erectile tissue?
Permanent changes occur. The corpora cavernosa stretches to accommodate cylinders, natural function is permanently lost, some circulation is preserved, and sensation is usually preserved through different pathways.

This FAQ section addresses the practical, personal, and technical questions that prospective patients commonly have but may be embarrassed to ask their surgeons directly.
Remember: the above is my opinion based on my research, when you have questions; ask your medical provider for the definitive answer.

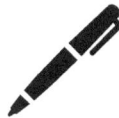

"In any moment of decision, the best thing you can do is the right thing, the next best thing is the wrong thing, and the worst thing you can do is nothing"

— Theodore Roosevelt

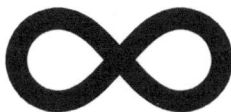

SUCCESS STORIES

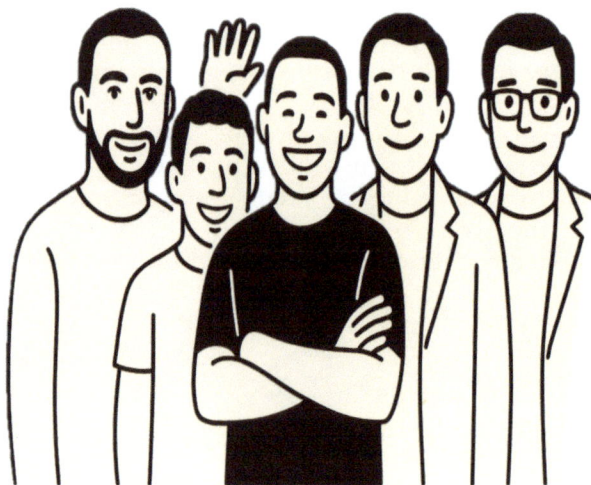

- **They Wished They Had Acted Sooner**
- **Their Life Has Improved!**

You Are Not Alone In Your Journey!

Chapter 11: Success Stories from Men Like Us

During my journey, I connected with several men who'd been though implant surgery. Their stories gave me hope that I want to share with you (all names changed, and details modified for privacy).

Michael, Age 62: A police officer whose ED started after a back injury led to nerve damage. "I thought my career in law enforcement meant I had to be tough about everything including this. Stupidest thing I ever believed. Getting my implant was like getting my confidence back on the job too. When you feel like a complete man again, it affects everything."

David, Age 45: Diagnosed with diabetes at 35, developed severe ED by 40. "My wife and I were trying to have a second child when my function completely disappeared. The implant not only restored our sex life but allowed us to conceive our daughter. She's now three, and I'm grateful every day that I didn't let pride stop me from getting help."

Robert, Age 58: A widower who thought his romantic life was over. "I met someone special two years after my wife passed, but I was terrified about intimacy. My implant gave me the confidence to pursue life again at an age when I thought that was impossible. We've been married for five years now."

James, Age 71: Retired military who waited too long to seek treatment. "I suffered for eight years because I was embarrassed to talk to a doctor about my penis. Eight years! I could have been having great sex all that time instead of avoiding my wife and feeling like less of a man. Don't make my mistake."

Carlos, Age 39: Developed ED after prostrate surgery for cancer. "Having cancer in my thirties was terrifying enough. Losing sexual function on top of that nearly broke me. My implant surgery was easier than my cancer treatment, and now I feel like I've beaten both diseases."

Tom, Age 66: A man whose marriage initially struggled but ultimately strengthened. "My wife was resistant to the idea of surgery at first. She thought it was 'unnatural' and worried about risks. After seeing how much happier and more confident I became, she admits it was the best decision we ever made. Our relationship is stronger now that it's been in decades."

What strikes me about all these stories is the common theme: every man wished he'd acted sooner. None regretted their decision. All found that their fears about surgery were worse than the reality. And most importantly, all reported that their lives improved in ways that extended far beyond the bedroom!

YOU are not alone on this journey! Thousands of men
have walked this path successfully before you!

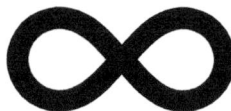

∞

Your Journey Continues Online

This book is just the beginning.
For ongoing support &
additional resources,
visit:

www.jayrichard.com

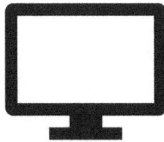

IN CONCLUSION

It's time for you to regain your sense of joy and intimacy.

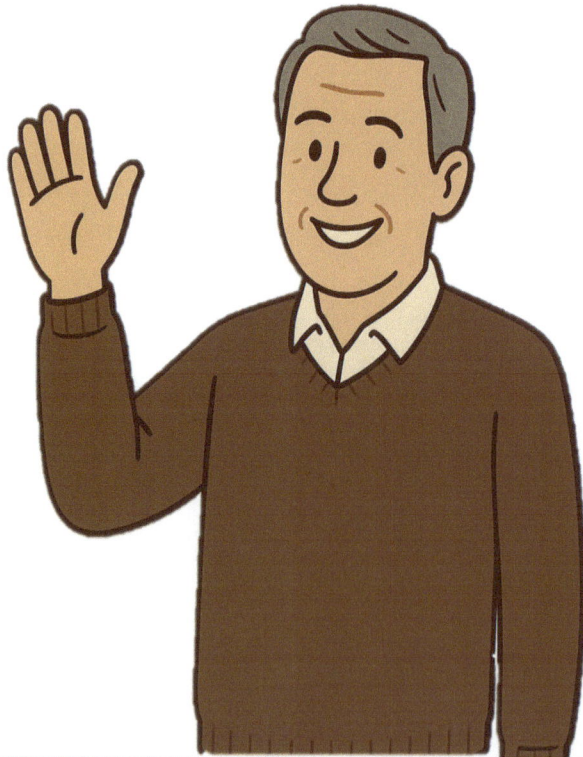

Conclusion: Your Path Forward

As I sit here writing this conclusion, two years after my penile implant surgery, I'm struck by how dramatically my life has changed. The man who once lay awake at 3 am, convinced his sex life was over, has been replaced by someone confident, satisfied, and grateful for the courage it took to seek advanced treatment.

The Journey We've Taken Together
Through these pages, we've traveled the complete journey from ED diagnosis to life-changing treatment.

We began with understanding, learning that ED is a common medical condition affecting millions of men, not a personal failing or sign of weakness.

We explored the progression, recognizing when first-line treatments like pills stop working and it's time to consider advanced options.

We examined the technology, understanding how modern penile implants work and which type might be best for your situation.

We navigated the practical decisions, from choosing a surgeon to understanding costs and insurance coverage.

We walked through the surgery experience, demystifying the process from preparation through recovery.

We addressed the often-forgotten partner perspective, recognizing that ED affects relationships, not just individuals.

We explored life after surgery, understanding the real-world experience of living with a penile implant.

Key Takeaways for Your Decision

If You're Still Deciding Whether to Pursue Treatment

Remember these truths: ED doesn't improve on its own, and waiting typically leads to worsening symptoms. You're not alone, as millions of men face this challenge successfully. Excellent treatments exist, as modern medicine offers highly effective solutions. Quality of life matters, and you deserve satisfying intimate relationships. The technology is sophisticated, with penile implants being reliable, safe, and effective.

Ask yourself these questions: How significantly is ED affecting my happiness and relationships? What would restored sexual confidence mean to my life? Am I ready to stop accepting a diminished quality of life? Do I have the support system needed for this journey? What would I regret more trying and facing temporary challenges, or never trying at all?

If You're Moving Forward with Treatment

Focus on these priorities: Choose an experienced surgeon, as this decision matters more than device brand. Understand all costs and plan financially for this investment in your future. Involve your partner to make this a shared journey when possible. Set realistic expectations by understanding what implants can and cannot do. Commit to the process, as recovery and adaptation take time and patience.

The Larger Message

This book isn't just about penile implants—it's about refusing to accept diminished quality of life when effective treatments exist. It's about having the courage to seek help for intimate health problems. It's about investing in your happiness and your relationships.

The principles apply beyond ED: Face health challenges directly rather than hoping they'll resolve on their own. Seek expert help when problems exceed your ability to solve them. Don't let embarrassment prevent you from getting needed medical care. Consider your partner in health decisions that affect your relationship. Invest in treatments that significantly improve quality of life.

A Personal Reflection

Looking back on my journey, I wish I had acted sooner. The years I spent hoping ED would improve on its own, trying various treatments halfheartedly, and avoiding the reality of my situation were years of unnecessarily diminished life quality.

What I learned: Courage is required, but the courage to seek help is far easier than the courage to keep living with the problem. Medical solutions exist for almost every health challenge, including intimate ones. Support is available from medical professionals, partners, and other men who've walked this path. The anticipation is worse than the reality, as fear of treatment often exceeds the actual experience. Life can be better than before, as treatment doesn't just restore function but often improves it.

For Partners Reading This

Your support, understanding, and encouragement can make the difference between treatment success and continued suffering. Remember that this affects you too, and you're not a bystander on this journey. Your feelings matter, and it's normal to have complex emotions about ED and its treatment.

You can help, as your support significantly impacts treatment success. Relationships can grow stronger, with many couples reporting better intimacy after successful ED treatment.

Professional help is available, so don't hesitate to seek counseling if needed.

The Broader Impact

When men successfully treat ED, the benefits extend far beyond the bedroom. Personal benefits include increased confidence in all life areas, reduced anxiety and depression, improved overall life satisfaction, and better physical and mental health. Relationship benefits encompass enhanced intimacy and communication, stronger partnership through shared challenges, increased relationship satisfaction, and better conflict resolution skills.

Societal benefits include reduced stigma through open discussion, increased awareness of treatment options, better support for other men facing similar challenges, and improved understanding of men's health issues.

Looking to the Future

The field of sexual medicine continues to advance rapidly. Future developments may include even more sophisticated implant technology, less invasive surgical techniques, improved materials and durability, better patient selection and outcomes, and expanded insurance coverage and accessibility.

For men considering treatment now, these advances mean even better options may be available when device replacement is eventually needed.

A Call to Action

If you're reading this book because you're struggling with ED, especially if pills have stopped working, I urge you to act.

Don't wait for the problem to get better on its own, because it won't.

Don't wait for a more convenient time, because there isn't one.

Don't wait for perfect circumstances, because they don't exist.

Don't wait for someone else to make the decision for you, because this is your choice.

Do Take These Steps:

Consult with a urologist specializing in sexual medicine.

Learn about all your treatment options.

Involve your partner in the decision-making process.

Understand the financial implications and plan accordingly.

Decide based on your goals and values.

Final Words of Encouragement

The decision to pursue advanced ED treatment, particularly penile implant surgery, isn't easy. It requires courage, commitment, and faith in medical technology and your surgical team. But for the thousands of men who make this choice each year, the results speak for themselves with over ninety percent patient satisfaction rates, dramatic quality of life improvements, restored sexual confidence and function, and enhanced relationships and overall happiness. You have the power to change your situation. The technology exists, qualified surgeons are available, and support systems are in place. The only question is whether you'll find the courage to take the first step.

Remember that you deserve to be happy and sexually fulfilled.

Help is available from qualified medical professionals. You're not alone on this journey. Success is not just possible, it's probable with proper treatment. The best time to act is now.

A Promise and a Challenge

I promise you this: if you have the courage to seek help, commit to the treatment process, and work with qualified medical professionals, your life can be dramatically better. Not just your sex life, but your overall confidence, happiness, and relationship satisfaction.

I challenge you to stop accepting less than the quality of life you deserve.

Stop letting ED steal another day, another month, another year from your happiness. The solutions exist—the question is whether you'll have the courage to pursue them.

Your journey to restored sexual health and renewed confidence starts with a single step: deciding that you deserve better.

Take That Step Today!

Remember: This book is your road-map, but every journey is unique.

Work with qualified medical professionals to develop the treatment plan that's right for your specific situation.

Your future self, and your partner, will thank you for having the courage to act.

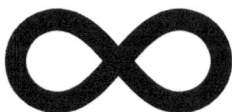

∞

Acknowledgments

This book wouldn't have been possible without the support, expertise, and encouragement of many people who contributed to both my personal journey and the creation of this resource.

To Dr. William Figlesthaler ("Dr. Fig"): Your surgical expertise, clear communication, and compassionate care transformed my life. Thank you for your patience with my questions, your skill in the operating room, and your ongoing support throughout this journey.

To my current partner: You're understanding and support during the most vulnerable period of my life gave me the strength to seek treatment and see it through to success. This journey was ours together.

To the men who shared their own experiences and provided encouragement when I needed it most. Your openness about this sensitive topic helped me feel less alone.

To future readers: May this book provide the information, encouragement, and hope you need to make the best decision for your situation and reclaim the quality of life you deserve.

To Donald J. Brown, whose strategic expertise and publishing guidance transformed this book from concept to professional publication. His understanding of both market dynamics and technical execution ensured this resource could reach the men who need it most. His dedication to quality and attention to detail elevated every aspect of this project.

ADDITIONAL RESOURCES

For support materials, and more information visit:

www.jayrichard.com

www.ingramcontent.com/pod-product-compliance
Lightning Source LLC
Chambersburg PA
CBHW040936030426
42335CB00001B/14